Nature's Medicine Cabinet

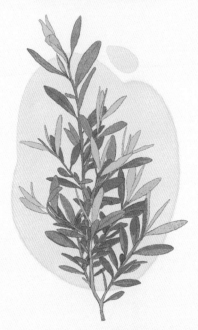

13-Digit ISBN: 978-1-40034-082-8
10-Digit ISBN: 1-40034-082-9

This book may be ordered by mail from the
publisher. Please include $5.99 for postage and
handling. Please support your local bookseller first!

Books published by Cider Mill Press Book
Publishers are available at special discounts for bulk
purchases in the United States by corporations,
institutions, and other organizations. For more
information, please contact the publisher.

Cider Mill Press Book Publishers
"Where good books are ready for press"
501 Nelson Place
Nashville, Tennessee 37214

cidermillpress.com

Typography: Fleur, Nave, Warnock Pro

Printed in Malaysia
24 25 26 27 28 OFF 5 4 3 2 1
First Edition

The information in this book is intended for educational purposes only and should not be considered
as medical advice. Herbal remedies can interact with medications and may not be suitable for everyone.
Always consult with a qualified healthcare professional before starting any new treatment, especially if
you are pregnant, nursing, have a medical condition, or are taking prescription medications. The author
and publisher are not responsible for any adverse effects or consequences resulting from the use of any
suggestions, preparations, or procedures discussed in this book.

NATURE'S MEDICINE & CABINET

Seasonal Remedies & Recipes for a Year of Botanical Wellness

MEAGAN VISSER

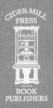

CIDER MILL
PRESS

BOOK
PUBLISHERS

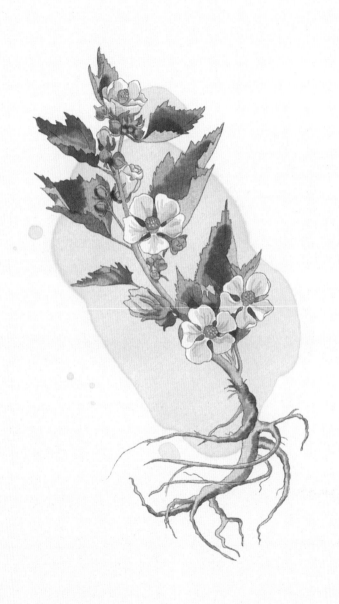

CONTENTS

FOREWORD

As a primary form of healthcare for centuries in cultures across the world, it's no surprise that herbalism has much to offer body, mind, and spirit—plants and humans have long formed a natural partnership. More and more, modern families are tapping into its potential as an effective addition to their wellness toolkit, whether for acute first aid needs or longer term wellness support.

Reaching for herbs in times of need can be both practical and empowering, and has the beautiful benefit of nurturing our connection with the natural world, be that with plantain and ground ivy growing in our lawns or St. John's wort and yarrow dancing in the summer meadows that draw our eye. Plant allies grow abundantly in our landscapes, are a vital part of the ecosystems of which we are part, and offer us the opportunity to connect with them throughout the seasons.

We are pleased to join herbalist Meagan Visser in celebrating her beautiful compilation, *Nature's Medicine Cabinet*. As a registered nurse with years of experience in herbalism, Meagan offers a pragmatic and thoughtfully considered approach to building a seasonal herbal apothecary for those seeking to support their family's wellness herbally.

Having had the pleasure of knowing Meagan for over a decade, we've watched her skillfully care for her family using herbal practices through many seasons as she has raised her four boys from infancy to adolescence. She shares much of these experiences, herbal recipes, and knowledge generously on her blog, *Growing Up Herbal*.

Our paths merged with Meagan's as she advanced her herbal education at the Herbal Academy, where she now teaches alongside us in numerous herbal programs. Meagan's insights, shaped by her medical background and her roles as a mother and herbalist, offer an abundance of support for those seeking to nurture their families by enlisting the power of herbs.

With the goal of sharing the recipes that have worked for her household over the years, Meagan expands so much of what she started on her blog to provide hands-on, practical guidance for getting started using herbs to support a range of daily wellness needs and first aid concerns. Arranged to provide recipes that work in synergy with and respond to the needs of each of the four seasons, this collection will help you gain familiarity with herbs as you build a personal herbal apothecary so you have what you need at the ready. You'll rest easy knowing what to turn to for everything from cuts, scrapes, and bruises to springtime allergies and autumn immune support.

Meagan has compiled this helpful guide to home herbalism, so you, too, can experience the joys and benefits of *growing up herbal*, no matter your age.

Best wishes in your herbal journey!

– **Jane Metzger and Amber Meyers,** Herbal Academy Co-Directors

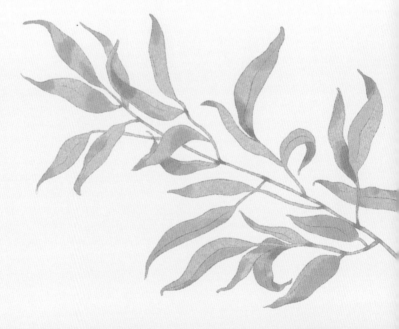

INTRODUCTION

Imagine having a medicine cabinet in your home filled with herbal preparations intended to support your and your family's wellness all year long—provided by nature!

I've done it, and I want to encourage and teach you how to do it too!

Herbalism has been the primary form of healthcare in my home for the past sixteen years, and apart from a handful of emergency situations, my family has been able to take charge of our own health naturally. This has not only saved us money and helped us avoid unnecessary medications and dependence on someone else where our health is concerned, but it has taught us to take personal responsibility for our own well-being, to work hard and stay dedicated to our vision, and to embrace a new way of thinking about health and wellness.

My herbal journey began sixteen years ago while I was pregnant with my first child. As a recent nursing school graduate, I was determined not to experience the many pregnancy complaints that were covered in my university women's health classes and clinicals—complaints that seemed all too common, yet could mostly be avoided with healthy lifestyle practices. After a fellow registered nurse gave me a book about herbs, a fire of empowerment was lit within me, and I dove headfirst into researching all things holistic and herbal, particularly where it related to supporting a healthy pregnancy. Little did I know that this would lead me down a path I would follow for many years to come, a path to embracing a practice that would change my life (and the life of my family) forever.

In the pages of this book, I will guide you on a journey through the seasons. I will introduce you to the various botanicals nature provides throughout the year, share some simple seasonal adjustments you can make to your diet and lifestyle, and bring some common seasonal ailments to your attention so you can be prepared for them ahead of time. I'm also sharing sixty herbal recipes—those that I use in my own home—that you can stock in your natural medicine cabinet to help you navigate these seasonal ailments as naturally as possible. Not only will you gain a deeper understanding of some basic herbal concepts, but you'll learn which supplies and ingredients to keep on hand, foraging practices you can follow if you want to harvest your own seasonal herbs, how to use herbs safely, and how to make a variety of herbal preparations.

By the end of this book, I hope to have encouraged you to approach your and your family's health and wellness from a natural perspective and to have inspired you to embrace seasonal herbalism in your home. From here, I want to support you on your herbal journey as you explore new paths and learn from other teachers. You never know where this practice will take you, but I can assure you that it will change your life for the better.

Before you venture any further, it is important to note that the information found in this book is for educational purposes only; it is not intended to diagnose, treat, cure, or prevent any disease or medical condition, and should not be used as a substitute for professional medical advice. While herbs have been the traditional medicine of choice for centuries, it is essential to consult with a qualified healthcare professional or an experienced clinical herbalist before incorporating herbs into your daily regimen, especially if you have pre-existing health conditions, are pregnant or nursing, or are taking pharmaceutical medications.

Alright, friend. Welcome to the wild and wonderful world of herbs—a place where ancient wisdom meets modern wellness! Get ready to unlock the transformative power of seasonal herbalism and embark on a path toward natural health and vitality.

AN ANCIENT PATH

Herbalism is a form of folk medicine, often referred to as "the people's medicine." It is rooted in ancient wisdom and practices that have been passed down from generation to generation. It is considered a traditional form of healthcare because it has been practiced for centuries by different cultures and communities worldwide.

Before the advent of modern medicine, people relied heavily on the resources available in their immediate surroundings, including various plants and herbs. They observed the effects of these botanicals on the body and developed a deep understanding of their properties and health applications.

Traditional herbalism is closely tied to indigenous communities' cultural and regional practices. It reflects their deep connection with nature and their ability to utilize local plants for wellness purposes. These traditional healing systems often incorporate holistic approaches that consider not only an individual's physical symptoms but also their emotional, mental, and spiritual well-being.

Herbal preparations and practices vary across different cultures, such as Traditional Chinese Medicine (TCM), Ayurveda, Native American herbalism, Celtic herbalism, African herbalism, Ashkenazi herbalism, and so on. Each of these traditions has their own unique theories, systems and diagnostic methods, preferred plants, and approaches to using herbs as part of their healing modalities.

Throughout the 1600s and 1700s, some of these herbal practices and traditions were brought to America. Along with Native American herbalism, these practices were primarily used by the common folk or those who didn't have access to doctors, as well as some wealthier individuals who'd had little success with the medical interventions practiced by orthodox physicians of the time. As herbalism's success and use began to spread, many nonorthodox physicians began to incorporate plants into their practices, eventually building upon the art and science of herbalism and tying these two worlds—traditional folk medicine and science-based medicine—together. In fact, herbalism was a common part of many medical practices up until the mid- to late 1800s.

However, due to the wide variety of medical theories and practices among physicians of the time, as well as the struggle for social, economic, philosophical, and political power, a medical standard of practice was created by the elite. This eventually led to a decrease in nonorthodox medical schools and, thus, less herbal practice among physicians. Because of this, the practice of traditional herbalism became obsolete for most people, except for those who kept it going in their homes and communities. Thankfully, an herbal resurgence occurred during the 1960s and 1970s with the back-to the-land movement, and today, herbalism once more plays a significant role in many communities as a primary or complementary form of healthcare. It is valued for its accessibility, affordability, and connection to nature; it acknowledges the wisdom of ancestral knowledge, respecting the interplay between humans and the plant world.

As for the future of herbalism, my heart longs to see individuals take their health into their own hands by incorporating natural, holistic practices into their daily lifestyles. I would love to see an herbalist in every home, once more making plants the first thing reached for in times of need, with each generation passing their botanical knowledge and wisdom down to the next. One day, I hope that knowing the plants that grow in one's backyard, the fields and meadows, or the forest is common knowledge. I also hope that stocking the home apothecary with seasonally harvested botanicals and filling one's natural medicine cabinet with handcrafted herbal tea blends, infused oils, salves, syrups, and tinctures are the norm. I yearn to see a shift in modern medical practice, one that allows physicians and other healthcare professionals to once again recommend and utilize herbs and more natural forms of medicine as an option for their patients, saving pharmaceuticals and more invasive interventions for when they are most needed.

ALLOWING THE SEASONS TO GUIDE YOU

One way to begin caring for yourself and your family more naturally is through the practice of seasonal herbalism.

Seasonal herbalism allows the cycles and rhythms of the year to dictate the plants you work with, your wellness focuses each season, and the types of herbal preparations you might want to keep in your natural medicine cabinet.

When you begin to think seasonally, the first thing you might focus on is the common ailments and conditions you and your family experience in different parts of the year. These ailments are highly individualized and can be influenced by your location, lifestyle choices, and family health.

Another way to take a seasonal approach to your health and wellness is through practicing bioregional herbalism, which is the study and use of plants that grow in your local area. As you become more attentive to seasonal cues, you might begin to notice the plants that grow around you and how they change throughout the seasons.

To get to know your local herbs a bit better, you can start by making a list of the plants you notice each season. You can then research the botanicals on your list to identify which ones are useful in herbalism, removing those that are not. It's also a good idea to see which botanicals are at risk of overharvesting; you'll want to remove these from your list or learn if they can be cultivated instead of wild-harvested. Next, you can begin to research each plant to identify how it's used, what its herbal actions and energetics are, any important safety or dosing information, and how to harvest and prepare it. It's also wise to list some alternate herbs that act similarly to the herb you are studying, as this will come in handy if you ever need to substitute one plant for another. Repeat this process for each botanical on your list, and after a while, you will know a lot about the herbs growing around you.

Whether you realize it or not, there are likely many plants available where you live. As you begin to make your list and see just how many useful plants there are, you may start to feel a bit overwhelmed, but let me assure you that you don't have to learn about all of the plants on your list at once. This process can take years, and you will constantly be adding new plants to your list. Pick a handful to start studying and using regularly and then add additional plants when you feel ready.

In the second half of this book, you will find lists of herbs that are commonly found and harvested in each season, as well as suggestions for seasonal lifestyle practices and wellness focuses you can incorporate into your lifestyle. Use these as a starting point on your seasonal herbal journey and see where it takes you.

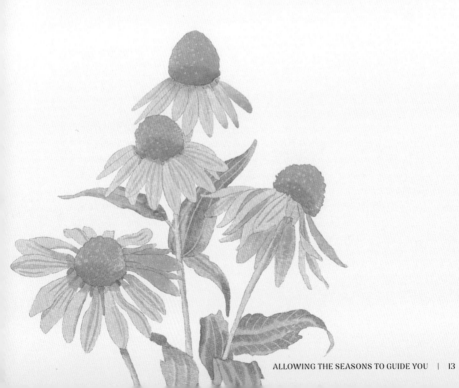

THE HOME
HERBALIST

As you embark on your journey as a home herbalist, there are a few things to consider before stocking your home apothecary with seasonal herbs or filling your natural medicine cabinet with herbal preparations for common seasonal ailments.

While this book isn't intended to be an herbal textbook, teaching you the art and science of herbalism as a whole, it will cover some important areas that will help guide you as you care for yourself and your family members naturally, including foundational herbal concepts, which supplies and ingredients to have on hand, how to identify and harvest seasonal botanicals, how to substitute one herb for another in a recipe, how to use herbs safely, and how to make a variety of herbal preparations.

If you're ready, let's begin.

Foundational Herbal Concepts

As mentioned previously, herbalism encompasses diverse cultural traditions from all over the world, is a combination of art and science, and combines traditional and modern practices. Yet, amid this medley, some foundational principles bring unity to all of herbalism's pieces in the twenty-first century.

Interconnection

All things are connected, from the cells and systems within the body to the larger, natural world of which we are a part. When something is out of balance, we must look inside and outside of ourselves to find possible causes and address these in both the inner and outer worlds. I'm reminded of the homeopathic wisdom of "like cures like"; we humans are a part of creation, and we can look to creation, whether to our local plants, to the sun or clean air and water, or to time outdoors in the mountains or at the ocean, to bring us back toward a state of balance.

A Body in Balance

The ultimate goal when using herbs for wellness is to bring the body back into equilibrium and keep it there for as long as possible. This is often achieved through using herbs that help activate, build, and/or cleanse the body so it can return to a balanced state of health. Activation is needed in times when the body is a bit sluggish and needs a boost or gentle nudge in the right direction. Building is needed when the body is in a weakened state, recovering from an ailment, or simply needs nourishment. Cleansing is needed when the body is burdened or loaded down by something that needs to be gently removed.

Use of Whole Plants

Herbalists generally use plant extracts made from whole plant material, which captures a wide range of phytochemicals found within the plant. These plant constituents work together synergistically to produce a variety of effects in the body. Using whole plants instead of isolated active ingredients helps reduce toxicity or side effects, making herbs quite safe for most individuals.

Use of Formulas

While it's good to use one herb at a time when you are getting to know a new plant—giving you time to familiarize yourself with how the plant works in your body—when using herbs for a specific condition, you can achieve greater results by combining plants together to create a formula. This formulation creates a synergistic effect, allowing the herbs to enhance, balance, support, and direct one another, which ultimately increases the formula's effectiveness.

An Individual Approach

Herbs are often matched to the individual and the specific symptoms of their condition to achieve the best results. Knowing how an herb works in the body, assessing how a condition is presenting itself in the individual, and then choosing the appropriate herbs to help bring the body back into a balanced state of health is key. It's important to note that herbalism is not a "set it and forget it" practice. It is quite common to make adjustments in herbal formulas and protocols along the way to better achieve the desired end result.

Now that you have an understanding of some of the principles herbalism is built upon, let's look at some things you'll need to have on hand to stock your home apothecary so you can care for yourself and your family naturally.

Sourcing Supplies & Ingredients

There are numerous ways to use herbs in your home throughout the season, but when it comes to using herbs for wellness purposes, the most common way to use them is through a variety of herbal preparations, such as teas, tinctures, salves, poultices, and more. Some of these preparations are made and used right away, and others are created and stored for later use. To make these herbal preparations, you will need to gather some basic supplies and ingredients, many of which you might already have in your home.

Here is a list of common kitchen and storage supplies, as well as some basic ingredients to have on hand so you are ready to make the seasonal recipes in the second half of this book. For items you don't already have on hand, try searching for them at local or online shops, thrift stores, garage sales, and flea markets, or borrow them from a friend or family member.

Supplies:

- Baking sheet
- Cheesecloth (unbleached)
- Coffee filters (unbleached)
- Coffee grinder
- Cotton/linen cloth or paper towels
- Cutting board
- Digital kitchen scale
- Electric mixer
- Eye wash cup
- Fine-mesh sieve
- Glass canning jars with lids (various sizes)
- Glass measuring cups or graduated cylinders
- Glass storage containers (various sizes)
- Gloves
- Heat-proof cups or mugs
- High-speed blender
- Immersion blender
- Juicer
- Knives
- Labels
- Measuring spoons
- Mixing bowls (various sizes)
- Natural waxed paper
- Pens, pencils, or markers
- Personal blender
- Saucepans (various sizes)
- Seed-warming mat
- Spoons
- Strainers
- Tins (various sizes)
- Toothpicks
- Water kettle

Ingredients:

- Activated charcoal
- Alcohol (40-95% ABV, such as brandy, whiskey, vodka, or grain alcohol)
- Aloe gel and juice
- Apple cider vinegar
- Arrowroot powder
- Baking soda
- Beeswax
- Bentonite clay
- Butters (cocoa or shea)
- Carrier oils (olive, coconut, sweet almond, etc.)
- Citric acid
- Cornstarch
- Essential oils
- Food-grade vegetable glycerin
- Herbs (fresh or dried)
- Hydrosols
- Maple syrup
- Menthol crystals
- Nut butter
- Raw honey
- Salt (sea, Celtic, Epsom, etc.)
- Seeds (flax and chia)
- Vitamin E oil
- Water (spring or filtered)

Once you have your supplies and ingredients on hand, you'll need to gather some herbs to make the preparations you want to stock in your natural medicine cabinet each season. Herbs can be sourced by purchasing, growing, or wildcrafting them.

Purchasing Dried Herbs

If you are new to using herbs, one of the simplest ways to source them is to purchase them from reputable local or online herb stores or suppliers. They are almost always dried, cut and sifted, and ready for use. Before purchasing, it's a good idea to ask where the plants were sourced, whether sustainable harvesting methods were used, and if the botanicals were tested for purity. Remember, you are taking plants from nature and putting them on and in your body, so asking these questions is not only important for your own overall wellness, but the sustainability and future supply of the plants as well.

Growing Herbs

Another way to source herbs is to grow them yourself. If you are new to growing herbs, it's a great idea to have a book about herb gardening on hand to use as a reference when starting your garden. You can also take a local or online class on the subject. You can even ask a friend with an herb garden for advice and see if they have any seeds they wouldn't mind sharing with you to help get your garden started.

If starting plants from seed isn't an option, you can purchase herb seedlings from local or online nurseries. Grocery stores will sometimes carry potted culinary herbs you can purchase and replant as well. Just be sure to look for organic varieties and suppliers that don't spray their plants with pesticides. You can also ask your herb gardening friends to share any extra perennial plants they've recently divided with you!

Wildcrafting Herbs

As you continue on your herbal journey, chances are you will learn how to identify more and more plants that grow in your area, whether in the forest, fields, or meadows. Wildcrafting plants can be a great way to gather herbs for free. It also allows you to play a bigger role in stewarding the land around you and helps you to connect with nature on a deeper level.

If you're interested in harvesting local plants, knowing how to properly identify plants and sustainably harvest them is essential. Many plant species have look-alike counterparts with significant differences in how they work in the body, such as yarrow (*Achillea millefolium*) and Queen Anne's lace (*Daucus carota*), not to mention deadly look-alikes like poison hemlock (*Conium maculatum*) and water hemlock (*Cicuta maculata*), all of which have white lacy flowers and feathery-looking leaves. Mistakenly harvesting the wrong plant can lead to ineffective formulas, potential poisoning, and even death, so precise plant identification is of the utmost importance if you plan to forage for your own herbs!

If you want to gather local plants, here are some tips and resources to help you along the way.

Plant Identification Tips

- Observe the physical characteristics of the plant by paying attention to key features, such as its leaf shape, arrangement, color, texture, flower structure, fruit or seed, stem, and overall growth habit.

- Use recommended field guides or reputable online resources that are specific to your region. These resources often provide descriptions, images, and distribution maps for plant identification.

- You may want to have a camera handy on your foraging trips to take clear photos of the plant in question. Be sure to take photos of the entire plant, as well as specific plant parts if necessary. These can come in handy when seeking outside help from a botanical expert.

- Pay attention to the natural environment where the plant is growing, including the type of soil, sun exposure, elevation, and surrounding vegetation. This information can help you narrow down possibilities during identification and help recreate the plant's preferred habitat if you decide to grow it in your garden.

- Some plants may exhibit different characteristics or undergo changes throughout the seasons, so it's a good idea to revisit the plant regularly throughout the year, taking note of the timing of flowering, fruiting, or other unique seasonal features, to assist with identification and the plant's growth cycle.

- If you are uncertain about a plant's identification, reach out to local botanical gardens, arboretums, or experienced herbalists or botanists who can provide guidance and help verify the identification. There are also some great plant identification groups on Facebook you can join as well.

- If you think you've identified a plant, it's wise to verify your findings using multiple reputable sources to ensure accuracy. Compare descriptions, images, and other distinguishing information to confirm the plant's identity.

Ethical Foraging Practices

- Avoid harvesting plants from protected areas, private property without permission, or locations that might be sprayed with chemicals or exposed to toxic residue.

- Do not harvest plants that are endangered or at risk of becoming endangered.

- To avoid overharvesting, harvest only what you will be able to process and use in one year's time, and take no more than 25 percent (or less, depending on the botanical) from a given plant stand.

- Minimize disturbance to the plant habitat and take care to harvest the plant in a way that allows the plant to regenerate if you are only taking a portion of it.

It's a good idea to maintain a foraging journal to document your observations, including details like location, date, plant characteristics, and any notes on potential uses or medicinal properties, for future reference and learning.

Keep in mind that proper plant identification takes time and practice. It can be helpful to engage with local plant identification groups, attend workshops or courses, or connect with experienced foragers who can provide hands-on guidance and share their knowledge with you.

Regardless of how you source your herbs, there are some common botanicals that can be helpful to keep on hand in your home apothecary. These plants are often used in a variety of herbal recipes and are a good starting place when sourcing herbs to keep in stock.

Herbs:

- **Astragalus**
  (*Astragalus mongholicus*) root
- **Burdock**
  (*Arctium lappa*) root
- **Calendula**
  (*Calendula officinalis*) flower
- **Chamomile**
  (*Matricaria chamomilla*) flower
- **Cleavers**
  (*Galium aparine*) aboveground
- **Cinnamon**
  (*Cinnamomum* spp.) bark
- **Comfrey**
  (*Symphytum officinale*) leaf
- **Dandelion**
  (*Taraxacum officinale*)
  leaf and root
- **Echinacea**
  (*Echinacea angustifolia*,
  E. purpurea) root
- **Elder** (*Sambucus nigra, S.
  canadensis*) flower and berry
- **Fennel**
  (*Foeniculum vulgare*) seed
- **Ginger**
  (*Zingiber officinale*) rhizome
- **Hawthorn**
  (*Crataegus* spp.) flower and
  berry
- **Lavender**
  (*Lavandula* spp.) flower bud
- **Licorice**
  (*Glycyrrhiza glabra*) root
- **Marshmallow**
  (*Althaea officinalis*) root
- **Mullein**
  (*Verbascum thapsus*) leaf
- **Nettle**
  (*Urtica dioica*) leaf
- **Oat**
  (*Avena sativa*) seed and straw
- **Peppermint**
  (*Mentha* x *piperita*) leaf
- **Plantain**
  (*Plantago* spp.) leaf
- **Raspberry**
  (*Rubus* spp.) leaf
- **Rose**
  (*Rosa* spp.) flower
- **Rosemary**
  (*Salvia rosmarinus*) leaf
- **Sage**
  (*Salvia officinalis*) leaf
- **Skullcap**
  (*Scutellaria lateriflora*)
  aerial parts
- **Thyme**
  (*Thymus vulgaris*) aerial parts
- **Tulsi**
  (*Ocimum tenuiflorum*) aerial
  parts
- **Valerian**
  (*Valeriana officinalis*) root
- **Yarrow**
  (*Achillea millefolium*) aerial
  parts

Making Substitutions

Once you've stocked your home apothecary with the supplies, ingredients, and herbs you want to keep on hand, you are ready to begin making seasonal herbal preparations to fill your natural medicine cabinet.

As you go about this process, you might come across an ingredient or herb in a recipe that you don't have on hand or simply don't want to use. When this happens, don't worry. You can always replace it with a suitable substitute.

Where substituting ingredients is concerned, you have plenty of options. However, it's important to remember that recipes may not turn out as originally intended when certain substitutions are made. For example, substituting vegan wax instead of beeswax in a salve can change the hardness, texture, and color of the final product, or substituting a dry sweetener for a liquid sweetener in a syrup can change the final flavor, texture, color, and possibly shelf-life of the final product. Therefore, it may take some ingredient research and trial and error to get the recipe as close to the original as possible.

Below, you will find a list of general ingredient substitutes you can make.

ORIGINAL INGREDIENT	SUBSTITUTE WITH
Alcohol	Food-grade vegetable glycerin
Apple cider vinegar	Any vinegar of your choice (red/white wine, rice wine, sherry, etc.)
Beeswax	Any wax of your choice (berry, caranuba, rice bran, soy, etc.)
Bentonite clay	Any clay of your choice (green, kaolin, pink, yellow, rhassoul, white, etc.)
Brandy	Any similar ABV alcohol of your choice (gin, rum, vodka, whiskey, etc.)
Cocoa butter	Any butter of your choice (avacado, kokum, mango, shea, etc.)
Cornstarch	Arrowroot powder

Honey	Any sweetener of your choice (coconut sugar, maple syrup/sugar, food-grade vegetable glycerin, stevia, unbleached and non-GMO cane sugar, etc.)
Olive oil	Any carrier oil of your choice (avocado, fractionated coconut oil, grapeseed, sweet almond, etc.)
Sea salt	Any salt of your choice (Celtic, Fleur de sel, Himalayan, etc.)

As for substituting herbs, you still have plenty of options, but you have to be a bit more strategic in choosing the right substitute herb if you want to achieve the same results as the original recipe intended.

To do this, you'll need to take the three foundational properties of the original herb into consideration before choosing a substitute herb. These three foundational herbal properties are tissue affinity, energetics, and actions.

Tissue Affinities

Tissue affinities are the tissues, organs, or body systems that an herb targets or affects. This might be the mucous membranes (or another type of tissue), the liver (or another specific organ), or the entire cardiovascular system (or other body system). Some herbs act primarily upon one tissue, while others affect multiple tissues throughout the body.

Peppermint (*Mentha* x *piperita*) leaf, for example, has a tissue affinity for the respiratory, digestive, and cardiovascular systems. We can get even more specific by noting that peppermint directly affects the smooth muscle tissue throughout each of these body systems. When looking for a substitute for peppermint, you will want to find another herb with an affinity for similar tissues.

Herbal Energetics

Herbal energetics are an herb's energy characteristics, which affect the tissues it has an affinity for in the body. According to Western herbalism, herbal energetics are fixed and unchanging and are associated with temperature, moisture, and tissue structure.

TEMPERATURE	MOISTURE	STRUCTURE
cooling to warming	moistening to drying	relaxing to toning

Herbal energetics can be quite subjective, and some herbalists have differing opinions when it comes to the energetic characteristics of certain plants. The energetics of a plant can often be determined through the senses, which is why it's so important to familiarize yourself with one plant at a time and get to know it well through regular use.

Using peppermint (*Mentha* x *piperita*) leaf again as an example, we can determine that this botanical has cooling, drying, and relaxing energetics. When looking for a substitute for peppermint, you will want to find another herb with similar energetics.

Herbal Actions

Herbal actions are the terms an herbalist uses to describe a plant's physiological effects on the body's tissues. These terms can be very generalized, such as "alterative," or quite specific, such as "lymphatic." However, at their core, herbs act on tissues by stimulating, relaxing, or toning the tissues. Herbs that stimulate work to increase the metabolic activity or function of the tissues. Herbs that relax work to decrease the metabolic activity or function of the tissues. Herbs that tone work to bring metabolic activity or function of the tissues back into a state of balance or equilibrium.

In our peppermint (*Mentha* x *piperita*) leaf example, we can do some research to find that this herb primarily relaxes the tissues thanks to the aromatic qualities of the plant's volatile oil content. This relaxing quality gives peppermint its herbal actions as an anodyne (eases pain), carminative (eases gas and bloating), diaphoretic (increases perspiration), febrifuge (cooling to the body), and spasmolytic (eases smooth muscle spasm). When substituting an herb for peppermint, you'll want to ensure the substitute works in a similar way within the body.

As you look over the recipes in the second half of this book, you will see many different herbs used throughout. Some herbs are included in multiple recipes, while others are specific to one or two recipes. If desired, feel free to substitute a more commonly used herb for a lesser-used herb to help simplify things on your end.

Now that you know how to source herbs and make substitutions when needed, let's look at how to use herbs safely.

Using Herbs Safely

While herbs are incredibly safe for most people, especially when compared to many pharmaceutical medications, they aren't always a fit for everyone at all times.

Because of this, it's essential to take the following things into consideration:

- A person's age and stage of life: for instance, young children, pregnant and/or nursing individuals, or older adults.

- Having a history of allergies, current chronic illnesses or health conditions, or current use of health supplements or pharmaceutical medications.

- Safety concerns specific to the herb, such as potential allergens or toxicities, interactions with certain supplements or pharmaceutical medications, or contradictions with particular health conditions.

Herbal Sensitivities and Allergies

One of the most common safety concerns when using herbs is the potential for unwanted side effects. Side effects are usually the result of sensitivities or allergies to a particular herb or family of herbs, but they can also be caused by improper usage and dosing.

Herbal sensitivities and allergies are most often mild. Rarely do life-threatening allergic reactions occur from herbs, but it pays to be mindful of potential herbal allergies, especially if a person has a history of allergies to food, plants, or medications.

Reactions due to herbal sensitivities or allergies often include hives or rashes on the skin, itching of the skin, throat, or eyes, watery eyes or a runny nose, and/or an upset stomach or diarrhea.

The most common herbal allergies are associated with plants in the Asteraceae (daisy) family, such as chamomile (*Matricaria chamomilla*), calendula (*Calendula officinalis*), echinacea (*Echinacea* spp.), yarrow (*Achillea millefolium*), etc., so it is important to test individual herbs for allergies before using them, especially plants in this family. Individuals with a history of severe allergic reactions should test for herbal allergies under the supervision of an experienced medical professional.

To test an herb for a potential allergy, follow these steps.

- Begin by rubbing the fresh herb on the inside of the wrist and waiting to see if a skin reaction occurs. If you only have access to the dried herb, soak it in a bit of warm water and rub the moistened herb on the skin first. If no reaction occurs, move on to the next step.
- Next, make a strong herbal infusion and drink 1 teaspoon (5 mL). Wait 30 minutes.
- If no reaction occurs, drink 1 tablespoon (15 mL). Wait another 30 minutes.
- If no reaction occurs, drink ½ cup (120 mL), and wait another 30 minutes.
- Finally, if no reaction occurs, try 1 full cup (240 mL).

If there is no reaction after following these steps, it's unlikely that you have an allergy to this herb.

Improper Herb Usage

Using an herb inappropriately can also lead to unwanted side effects. Inappropriate usage can include using the wrong plant for a given situation (e.g., using a drying herb when the tissues are already dry), taking too high a dose or using an herb for too long, using a potent herb when a gentle one is sufficient, or even using an herb while taking health supplements or pharmaceutical medications. In addition, the use of certain herbs should be avoided in small children, pregnant and nursing individuals, and older adults due to their potency and/or herbal actions within the body.

It is for these reasons that it's essential to do proper research on a new herb or to seek the advice of an experienced herbalist or medical professional with herbal training to determine if an herb is appropriate for you. If you come across an herb that isn't a fit for you in a recipe, feel free to substitute another herb in its place.

Alcohol Tinctures and Children

Another common herbal safety concern, particularly for parents, is whether or not it's okay to give alcohol tinctures or other alcohol-based preparations, like cordials and elixirs, to children.

Many health experts recommend avoiding the use of alcohol during childhood because children are smaller, making it easier to over-consume alcohol, and have less developed metabolic pathways than adults, which impacts how efficiently alcohol can be metabolized by the body. While the topic of limiting alcohol for minors is generally centered around consuming larger amounts of alcohol in beverages rather than the small amounts one would receive in herbal preparations, pharmaceutical medications, and even fermented foods, some would argue that alcohol in any amount is unsafe.

In herbalism, alcohol is a commonly used solvent. It extracts a wide range of plant constituents, is quickly absorbed and fast-acting, and helps extend the shelf life of herbal preparations. Many herbalists, including those with medical backgrounds and extensive training, are not opposed to using alcohol tinctures or other alcohol-based preparations when working with most children, particularly when the benefits of an alcohol-based preparation outweigh the concerns.

The negative effects of alcohol are often related to the overall amount consumed. While there is no safe limit established for alcohol, it is generally suggested that adult males consume no more than 3 fl oz (90 mL) of 40% ABV per day and adult females consume no more than 1.5 fl oz (45 mL) of 40% ABV per day to avoid health problems that can occur from excessive alcohol use.

In herbalism, most dosage suggestions are weight-based and generally calculated for a 150-pound adult. For example, if a suggested adult tincture dose with 40% ABV is 50-100 drops (2.5-5 mL) three times a day, then you can see that the high end of the daily dosage comes to 300 drops (15 mL) and does not exceed the upper limit of alcohol for males or females.

For anyone above or below 150 pounds, especially children,, the suggested dose needs to be recalculated based on the individual's weight to ensure they are receiving a safe and proper dose for their body size. This is true for alcohol tinctures but also for other herbal preparations, such as teas, pastilles, and syrups. To do this, you can follow Clark's Rule.

CLARK'S RULE (WEIGHT-BASED)

Individual's weight in pounds, divided by 150, then multiplied by the suggested dose

Example: Suggested dose of 50-100 drops (2.5-5 mL) 3x/day recalculated for a 27-pound two-year-old child
  Lower dosage limit: 27 ÷ 150 = .18 x 50 (2.5 mL) = 9 (0.5 mL)
  Upper dosage limit: 27 ÷ 150 = .18 x 100 (5 mL) = 18 (1 mL)
  Child's final suggested dosage: 9-18 drops (0.5-1 mL) 3x/ day

As you can see, calculating alcohol-based herbal preparation dosages based on an individual's weight regardless of age is the safest way to ensure the individual doesn't exceed the recommended limit for daily alcohol consumption.

If you feel comfortable using alcohol tinctures with children, you can add the tincture to a small amount of water, juice, or smoothie to mask the flavor and make them easier to take. You can also place the tincture dose in a small amount of just-boiled water for fifteen minutes to encourage alcohol evaporation, thus reducing the total amount of alcohol consumed. Lastly, you can make and use smaller-ratio tinctures, such as 1:2 or 1:3, to decrease the total amount of alcohol present in each dose.

While tinctures are a wonderful preparation and have their place in the natural medicine cabinet, you don't have to use tinctures or any other alcohol-based preparation if you don't feel comfortable. If you want to completely avoid alcohol in your natural medicine cabinet, you have a couple of options.

For herbal preparations that call for alcohol, such as cordials, elixirs, and tinctures, you can use food-grade vegetable glycerin in place of the alcohol in the recipe. Glycerin is a sweet-tasting liquid that extracts some of the same plant constituents as alcohol, making it a good option as an alcohol-free substitute. Not only that, but it's shelf-stable for one to three years and tastes great, so your kids won't mind taking it.

Another idea for those who want to avoid alcohol with children is to rework the recipe, turning it from an alcohol-based preparation into a water-based preparation, such as tea or syrup. Teas and syrups are wonderful preparations for children as they are palatable, easily absorbed, and easy to administer. To change the preparation type, identify any herbs in the recipe that are ideally extracted in alcohol and replace them with substitutes that are best extracted in water if need be. Most herbs that are tinctured are also used in water-based preparations, so chances are you won't have to substitute anything here, but it is something to keep in mind. This will help your child—or anyone who wants to avoid alcohol—to get the same benefits and results from the recipe in a form that feels safe to you.

Incorporating Essential Oils into Herbal Preparations

Incorporating essential oils into herbal preparations can enhance their overall benefits, but safety is paramount, especially when considering proper dilution. Essential oils are highly concentrated substances, and, according to Robert

Tisserand, renowned aromatherapist and author of *Essential Oil Safety*, they should always be diluted before application to the skin or inclusion in herbal products.

The appropriate dilution depends on the age of the user and the intended use.

For adults, a 1-2% dilution is typically recommended for general or long term use or use on a large surface area of the body, and a 5-10% dilution for acute or short term use or use on a small surface area of the body.

For children, much lower concentrations are necessary to avoid irritation or adverse reactions. Robert Tisserand suggests the following essential oil dilution guidelines for children:

- Infants (0-3 months): 0.1-0.2%
- Babies (3-24 months): 0.25-0.5%
- Toddlers and young children (2-6 years): 1-2%
- Older children (6-15 years): 1.5-3%

These dilutions ensure that essential oils are used appropriately for a child's age and sensitivity.

Essential oils included in recipes in the second half of this book are calculated for adult use. If you are making a recipe for a child, you will need to recalculate the essential oil dilution for the appropriate age of your child.

When to Seek Advanced Help

While herbs are known as "the people's medicine," they have their limitations.

Herbal preparations are whole-plant extracts that work to bring the body back into a state of balance, not lab-formulated pharmaceuticals that use synthetic or isolated compounds and work in a targeted or direct manner to produce a specific end result. This means that herbs might take some time to bring about the desired results you are seeking, or you may have to adjust the herbs you are using along the way to achieve better results. There may also be times when our efforts are not enough, and we need to seek the help of an experienced herbalist or medical professional. Depending on where you are on your herbal journey and the education and experience you have acquired thus far, you may want to seek advanced help for any of the following situations:

- An acute condition that doesn't improve or begins to worsen after a few days.
- A chronic condition that is beyond your scope of knowledge and ability.
- Working with an individual taking pharmaceutical medications.
- Working with a pregnant or nursing individual.

Seeking help can be a good thing and is something to be expected on this journey. We all need a second opinion from time to time, and pursuing guidance from someone more knowledgeable and experienced, whether that's another herbalist or a medical professional, will only make you a better and wiser herbalist in the long run.

Now that you have a home apothecary full of supplies, ingredients, and herbs that nature has provided, and you know how to use botanicals safely, it's time to start filling your natural medicine cabinet with herbal preparations that will support you throughout the coming seasons.

Making Herbal Preparations

There are many different types of herbal preparations you can make, such as infusions, decoctions, syrups, tinctures, glycerites, pastilles, lozenges, succi, etc., and there are an equal number of ways to make each preparation. Every herbalist has their preferred method, but the two most common ways to make herbal preparations are the folk method (also known as the simpler's method) and the mathematical method (also known as the weight-to-volume or ratio method).

The folk method is great for beginners because all ingredients are estimated, and very little math and few tools for precise measurements are required. In this method, measurements are given as parts, which offers flexibility in determining the overall batch size of a preparation. A part can be any unit of measurement you wish, such as a teaspoon, tablespoon, cup, ounce, pound, gram, milliliter, etc., as long as you use the same unit consistently throughout the recipe.

You may choose a cup for your part when making a large batch of tea, a tablespoon for your part when making a small batch of herb-infused oil, or 15 mL for the part when blending tinctures together to create a formula.

For example, if a tea or infusion recipe calls for 2 parts of a certain herb, and you are using a cup as your part, then you'll measure out 2 cups of that herb. If it calls for a ½ part of another herb, you'll measure ½ cup for that herb.

The other option is the mathematical method. This method is great for those who like a consistent recipe to follow, ensuring the end product turns out the same each time it's made. While the mathematical method can seem more complicated at first because it requires precise weights and measurements, the consistency it provides where dosing is concerned is well worth the effort.

When measuring ingredients for herbal recipes, liquid ingredients, such as carrier oils and honey, must be measured by volume (fluid ounces, milliliters), whereas dry items like beeswax and plant material, must be measured by weight (ounces, grams). Having a good digital kitchen scale and a set of glass measuring cups or graduated cylinders will help you accurately measure your ingredients.

For example, when making an herb-infused oil, you may measure 4 fl oz (120 mL) of carrier oil and weigh out .8 oz (20 g) of your chosen herb to create a potent herbal oil.

That said, I have formulated all the recipes in the second half of this book to be potent, effective, and easy for a beginner to follow.

You will find that most tea and tincture blends, as well as a few other herbal preparations, follow the folk method and call for measurements in parts to give you the option to control your batch size. I have used the mathematical method for all other recipes, including both imperial and metric measurements to make it easy for my American and international friends. To simplify things even further for my American friends and those not interested in weighing everything, I've also included volume estimates for dry ingredients using teaspoons, tablespoons, and cups. You're welcome!

While each recipe includes easy measurements and detailed directions, there are two types of herbal preparations—herb-infused oils and tinctures/glycerites—that give you some options in your preparation methods.

Herb-Infused Oils

Herb-infused oils are great preparations to have in the natural medicine cabinet. They can be used as is or turned into ointments, salves, and balms.

Over the years, I have found the most success in using heat to speed up the extraction process rather than using the traditional four-week room temperature maceration method. There are two simple ways to do this: the slow-heat method and the quick-heat method. Both of these methods are effective on their own, but each requires a different amount of time and attention.

The slow-heat method utilizes a seed-warming mat to keep the oil and herb combination warm for two weeks. Seed-warming mats are perfect heat sources for infused oils because they're waterproof, maintain a 70–85° F (21–29° C) temperature, and can be left on safely for extended periods of time. This method is primarily hands-off during this time, so it's an excellent method to use if you're not in a hurry to use the herb-infused oil.

Slow-Heat Herb-Infused Oil

- Begin by combining your carrier oil and dried herb in a clean, dry glass canning jar. (For a better extraction, grind the dried herbs in a coffee grinder before combining them with the oil.) Place a piece of natural waxed paper between the jar and the lid to help prevent any chemical coating or corrosion on the lid from coming into contact with the contents inside the jar, and label the jar with the name of the herb and oil used, as well as the finish date.

- Next, place the jar on a seed-warming mat for two weeks. Be sure to gently shake the jar every day or two to keep the contents mixed up inside, as this will help give you a better extraction. If you find that it's hard to maintain a minimum temperature of 70° F (21° C), you can lay a towel over the jar and seed mat to hold more heat in.

- When two weeks have passed, place a fine-mesh sieve (lined with a few layers of cheesecloth to remove plant material, if you wish) over a clean, dry glass container and carefully pour the mixture through it. Press the herbs with the back of a spoon (or gather the edges of the cheesecloth to create a bundle and gently squeeze) to extract as much liquid as possible. You can double strain the decanted liquid once more through a fine-mesh sieve lined with an unbleached coffee filter to further remove fine particles if you wish. Compost the used plant material.

- Reserve the finished herb-infused oil in a clean, labeled glass storage container in a cool, dark location for up to twelve months before making a fresh batch.

Quick-Heat Herb-Infused Oil

If you find yourself in a rush for an herb-infused oil, the quick-heat method is for you. This method utilizes the stovetop or crockpot to keep the oil and herb combination warm for 4–8 hours. Unlike the slow-heat method, this method is very hands-on because the temperature of the stovetop and crockpot is much higher and requires more maintenance and a watchful eye.

- Begin by combining your carrier oil and dried herb in a clean, dry glass canning jar. (For a better extraction, grind the dried herbs in a coffee grinder before combining them with the oil.) Place a piece of natural waxed paper between the jar and the lid to help prevent any chemical coating or corrosion on the lid from coming into contact with the contents inside the jar, and label the jar with the name of the herb and oil used, as well as the finish date.

- Next, place a few canning jar lids on the bottom of a saucepan or crockpot, set the sealed jar on the canning lids, and add enough room-temperature water to the saucepan or crockpot so that the water rises to the same level as the oil and herbs inside the jar (or within an inch of the top of the saucepan or crockpot). This will create a water bath–like environment for the herb-infused oil.

- Place the saucepan on the stovetop over low heat or turn the crockpot to a warm or low setting to bring the water to a simmer. As the water temperature rises, remove the lid from the herbal oil and use a digital thermometer to keep an eye on the temperature of the oil inside the jar. Once it reaches 120° F (49° C), set a timer for 4–8 hours. During this time, it's important to keep the oil temperature between 120-140° F (49-60° C), so you may need to turn the heat off and on to maintain this temperature or keep the oil from getting too hot. You'll also want to keep an eye on the water level inside the saucepan or crockpot to be sure it hasn't evaporated as well. If the water begins to get low, carefully remove the jar of herbal oil and add more hot water from the tap to bring the level back up before carefully placing the jar of herbal oil back into the water.

- When 4–8 hours have passed, carefully remove the jar from the water bath and allow it to cool slightly. Place a fine-mesh sieve (lined with a few layers of cheesecloth to remove plant material, if you wish) over a clean, dry glass container and carefully pour the mixture through it. Press the herbs with the back of a spoon (or gather the edges of the cheesecloth to create a bundle and gently squeeze) to extract as much liquid as possible. You can double strain the decanted liquid once more through a fine-mesh sieve lined with an unbleached coffee filter to further remove fine particles if you wish. Compost the used plant material.

- Reserve the finished herb-infused oil in a clean, labeled glass storage container in a cool, dark location for up to twelve months before making a fresh batch.

An 8-hour infusion is ideal, as this time frame allows for better extraction of the herbal constituents into the oil, but keeping the oil at that temperature for that amount of time can be difficult, so 4 hours is sufficient to produce a good quality oil. To determine if an oil is ready, you might pay attention to the color and scent of the oil. If it takes on a deeper color (depending on the color of the plant material—not all herbs produce colored oils) and begins to smell like the herb, then you know some extraction has taken place.

Herbal Tinctures and Glycerites

Tinctures are another wonderful herbal preparation to have on hand in the natural medicine cabinet. Not only are they potent, convenient to use, and long-lasting, but they can also be combined to create endless formulas to meet a variety of needs. Tinctures can be made using the folk method or the mathematical method.

Folk method tinctures are simple and easy to make, and they are the perfect tincture method for beginners. They require very little math or precise measurements, as all ingredients are estimated.

While folk tinctures have their merits, the downside is that they lack the standardization needed to create consistency from batch to batch, which means potency and, therefore, dosage will vary from batch to batch. While it's best practice to weigh the amount of herb used in a tincture to help you determine the proper daily dosage for each batch, a general dosage guide for folk tinctures is to use one drop of a 50% ABV tincture for every two pounds of body weight. You will then need to pay attention to how the tincture makes you feel or take note of noticeable improvements (or lack thereof) in your symptoms after using the tincture for a few days before titrating your daily dosage up or down based on your results.

Folk Tinctures

- Begin by filling a clean, dry glass canning jar half full of dried herbs or completely full of fresh herbs. Your plant material should be small, so be sure to garble, chop, or grind larger plant parts into smaller parts for better extraction. Weigh the plant material using a digital kitchen scale, so you know exactly how many grams of herb is in the final tincture.

- Add enough alcohol of your choice to cover the plant material completely. Fresh herbs are generally tinctured with 70% or higher alcohol by volume (ABV) and should be covered with 1 inch of alcohol. Dried herbs are generally tinctured with 40-60% ABV and should be covered with 2–3 inches (5–8 centimeters) of alcohol as the plant material will expand after soaking up some of the liquid. If you are tincturing dried herbs, check back after 24 hours to see if you need to add more alcohol to ensure there is at least an inch of liquid above the plant material. All plant material should be completely covered by 1 inch (2.5 centimeters) of alcohol during the entire maceration process, as any herb above the surface of the alcohol could begin to decompose or mold.

- Place a piece of natural waxed paper between the jar and the lid to help prevent any chemical coating or corrosion on the lid from coming into contact with the contents inside the jar.

- Label the jar with the name and total weight of the herb used, as well as the type of alcohol and ABV used. Give it a shake to make sure the contents are thoroughly mixed, and place it in a dark location for 4–6 weeks. Check it every couple of days to shake it again and see if the alcohol needs to be topped off a bit due to the herb's expansion.

- When 4–6 weeks have passed, place a fine-mesh sieve (lined with a few layers of cheesecloth to remove plant material, if you wish) over a clean, dry glass container and carefully pour the mixture through it. Press the plant material with the back of a spoon (or gather the edges of the cheesecloth to create a bundle and squeeze) to extract as much liquid from the plant material as possible. Compost the used plant material.

- If you wish, you can strain the liquid once more through a fine-mesh sieve lined with an unbleached coffee filter to further remove any fine particles. Alternatively, you can cover the jar and let it sit on the counter overnight, allowing any remaining herb sediment to settle at the bottom. In the morning, the clear, sediment-free liquid can then be carefully poured off the top. Removing as much sediment from the final tincture as possible helps to further extend the tincture's shelf life.

- Reserve the finished tincture in a labeled clean, glass storage bottle in a cool, dark location for 3–5 years before making a fresh batch.

Mathematical Tinctures

Mathematical tinctures can seem more complicated at first because they require you to research the correct alcohol percentage for the herb you are tincturing and to use precise ratios, weights, and measurements for ingredients. However, they produce a consistent end product each time they are made, which standardizes potency from batch to batch and makes dosing more precise.

- Begin by choosing the herb-to-solvent ratio you would like to use. Ratios tell you how much herb by weight and solvent (alcohol) by volume is in the final tincture. For example, a 1:4 tincture means for every 1 part herb by weight, 4 parts solvent by volume are used. The part you use can be weighed in ounces (oz) or grams (g) or measured in fluid ounces (fl oz) or milliliters (mL), depending on your measurement preferences. Fresh herbs are generally tinctured at a 1:2 or 1:3 ratio, whereas dried herbs are generally tinctured at a 1:3, 1:4, or 1:5 ratio, depending on the size of the plant part being tinctured. Ratios also affect the tincture dosage. The smaller the ratio, the more concentrated the tincture and, therefore, the smaller the dose. The larger the ratio, the less concentrated the tincture and, therefore, the larger the dose.

- Next, determine the percentage of alcohol required for the herb you are tincturing. Fresh herbs are generally tinctured with 70% or higher ABV, while dried herbs are generally tinctured with 40-60% ABV. For example, fresh dandelion (*Taraxacum officinale*) root might be tinctured at a 1:2 ratio with 70% ABV, whereas dried dandelion (*Taraxacum officinale*) leaf might be tinctured at a 1:5 ratio with 40% ABV. Fluffy plant material, such as calendula (*Calendula officinalis*) flower or mullein (*Verbascum thapsus*) leaf, might need to be tinctured at a 1:10 ratio so there is enough alcohol to cover the plant material.

- Finally, calculate how much herb or solvent is needed to make your tincture. While we Americans are used to the imperial system of measurement, the metric system is quite a bit easier to use where ratio tinctures are concerned, so that is the system we will use. There are two ways to do this. First, you can weigh out how much plant material you want to tincture, then multiply this number by the solvent portion of the suggested ratio for the herb you are using. For example, if you want to make a 1:5 peppermint (*Mentha* x *piperita*) leaf tincture, and you have 25 g of plant material, you would multiply 25 by 5 to find that you will need a total of 125 mL alcohol for the tincture. Alternatively, you can decide how much total volume of tincture you'd like to make and then divide this number by the herb portion of the suggested ratio for the herb you are using. For example, if you want to make a 4-ounce bottle of peppermint (*Mentha* x *piperita*) leaf tincture, and you have 120 mL of alcohol, you will need to divide 120 mL by 5 to find that you will need a total weight of 20 g of peppermint leaf for the tincture.

- Now that you have calculated and written down all of these numbers, you are finally ready to make your tincture! Using a digital kitchen scale, weigh the appropriate amount of herb you will need and place it in a clean glass canning jar. Your plant material should be small, so be sure to garble, chop, or grind larger plant parts into smaller parts for better extraction.

- Next, measure the appropriate amount of solvent (alcohol) using a glass measuring cup or graduated cylinder and pour it over the plant material. The herb should be submerged in the liquid throughout the entire extraction process, as any herb above the surface of the alcohol can begin to decompose or mold. If you find that there isn't enough solvent to cover all of the plant material, you will need to add more solvent until you have enough to sufficiently cover the herb. This will increase your ratio and change your final dose, so be sure to keep track of any additional alcohol you end up using.

- Place a piece of natural waxed paper between the jar and the lid to help prevent any chemical coating or corrosion on the lid from coming into contact with the contents inside the jar.

- Label the jar with the name and total weight of the herb used, as well as the type of alcohol and ABV used. Give it a shake to make sure the contents are thoroughly mixed, and place it in a dark location for 4–6 weeks. Check it every couple of days to shake it again and see if the alcohol needs to be topped off a bit due to the herb's expansion.

- When 4–6 weeks have passed, place a fine-mesh sieve (lined with a few layers of cheesecloth to remove plant material, if you wish) over a clean, dry glass container and carefully pour the mixture through it. Press the plant material with the back of a spoon (or gather the edges of the cheesecloth to create a bundle and squeeze) to extract as much liquid from the plant material as possible. Compost the used plant material.

- If you wish, you can strain the liquid once more through a fine-mesh sieve lined with an unbleached coffee filter to further remove any fine particles. Alternatively, you can cover the jar and let it sit on the counter overnight, allowing any remaining herb sediment to settle at the bottom. In the morning, the clear, sediment-free liquid can then be carefully poured off the top. Removing as much sediment from the final tincture as possible helps to further extend the tincture's shelf life.

- Reserve the finished tincture in a labeled glass storage bottle in a cool, dark location for 3–5 years before making a fresh batch.

Glycerites

Alcohol-free tinctures are often referred to as glycerites. These preparations are made similarly to tinctures, only using food-grade vegetable glycerin in place of alcohol as the solvent. Glycerin is a clear, sweet-tasting liquid that does not affect blood sugar levels, and it's a great solvent for those who don't like the taste of alcohol tinctures or want to avoid alcohol altogether. It extracts some of the same plant constituents as alcohol and has a shelf-life of 1–2 years. Glycerin is sourced from coconut, palm, or soybean oils, so it's important to purchase a sustainably harvested, non-GMO (genetically modified organism) variety from a reputable source.

To make an herbal glycerite, you will follow the exact same steps as the folk or mathematical tincture methods above, only instead of using alcohol as the solvent, you will use vegetable glycerin. If you are working with fresh herbs, you'll need to use 100% glycerin, as the fresh plant material already contains water. If you are working with dried herbs, you will need to use a 60% glycerin solution (4 parts water to 6 parts glycerin). This will allow you to extract both the water- and alcohol-soluble constituents from the plant material.

Glycerites are best prepared when heat is used during the maceration period, as heat helps to break the hydrogen bonds between the glycerin molecules, allowing it to better extract the plant constituents. You can do this just as you would if you were making an herb-infused oil, following either the slow-heat method, which utilizes a seed-warming mat, or the quick-heat method, which utilizes a crock pot or saucepan.

Glycerites can be more difficult to strain than tinctures as the glycerin is quite thick and viscous. Straining the liquid through a fine-mesh sieve lined with a layered cheesecloth while it is still warm can make the job easier, but be careful not to burn yourself. It can be a good idea to wear gloves to protect your hands from the heat!

Herbal glycerites are also dosed the same as tinctures. You can take them directly in the mouth, mix them with a small amount of water or juice, or add them to a smoothie or cup of tea.

Most of the tincture recipes in this book call for combining individual herbal tinctures using "parts," so you can make whatever size batch you wish. Not only that, but each herb has a certain percentage of alcohol that best extracts the constituents from the plant material; therefore, it is best to tincture herbs individually and later combine them into a formula. If you want to avoid alcohol, you can make individual herbal glycerites from herbs that are suitably extracted in glycerin and then combine them together to make the formula instead.

Tinctures (and their suggested alcohol percentage) to make ahead of time include:

Spring

- Chamomile (*Matricaria chamomilla*) flower - (40%)
- Cinnamon (*Cinnamomum* spp.) bark - (60%)
- Dandelion (*Taraxacum officinale*) root - (40-60%)
- Echinacea (*Echinacea angustifolia*) root** - (40%)

- Fennel (*Foeniculum vulgare*) seed - (40%)
- Licorice (*Glycyrrhiza glabra*) root - (30%)
- Orange (*Citrus* spp.) peel - (70%)
- Sage (*Salvia officinalis*) leaf - (40%)
- Yarrow (*Achillea millefolium*) aerial parts - (40%)

Summer

- Arnica (*Arnica* spp.) flower+ - (60%)
- Blue vervain (*Verbena hastata*) aerial parts - (40%)
- Cayenne (*Capsicum annuum*) fruit - (25%)
- Clove (*Syzygium aromaticum*) bud - (70%)

- Echinacea (*Echinacea angustifolia*) root** - (40%)
- Ginger (*Zingiber officinale*) rhizome - (40%)
- Grindelia (*Grindelia* spp.) flower bud - (70%)
- Lavender (*Lavandula* spp.) flower bud - (70%)

- Licorice (*Glycyrrhiza glabra*) root - (30%)
- Oregon grape (*Berberis aquifolium*) root** - (40%)
- Peppermint (*Mentha x piperita*) leaf - (40%)
- Plantain (*Plantago* spp.) leaf - (30%)

Autumn:

- California poppy (*Eschscholzia californica*) aboveground parts - (60%)
- Kava (*Piper methysticum*) root** - (60%)
- Lavender (*Lavandula* spp.) flower bud - (70%)

Winter

- Anise (*Pimpinella anisum*) seed - (40%)
- Chamomile (*Matricaria chamomilla*) flower - (40%)
- Echinacea (*Echinacea angustifolia*) root** - (40%)
- Goldenseal (*Hydrastis canadensis*) root tincture** - (60%)
- Hawthorn (*Crataegus* spp.) berry - (40%)
- Lemon balm (*Melissa officinalis*) aerial parts - (40%)
- Licorice (*Glycyrrhiza glabra*) root - (30%)
- Osha (*Ligusticum porteri*) root* - (70%)

- Skullcap (*Scutellaria lateriflora*) aerial parts - (40%)
- Willow (*Salix alba*) bark - (25%)
- Witch hazel (*Hamamelis virginiana*) bark - (40%)
- Wood betony (*Betonica officinalis*) aerial parts - (50%)

- Sage (*Salvia officinalis*) leaf - (40%)
- Valerian (*Valeriana officinalis*) root - (60%)
- Yarrow (*Achillea millefolium*) aerial parts - (40%)

- Passionflower (*Passiflora incarnata*) aerial parts - (40%)
- Rose (*Rosa* spp.) petal - (50%)
- Skullcap (*Scutellaria lateriflora*) aerial parts - (40%)
- Tulsi (*Ocimum tenuiflorum*) aerial parts - (25%)
- Usnea (*Usnea* spp.) lichen* - (50%)
- Valerian (*Valeriana officinalis*) root - (60%)
- White pine (*Pinus strobus*) needle - (50%)
- Wild cherry (*Prunus serotina*) bark - (40%)

+ external use only

***** **sustainably sourced**

****** **cultivated source**

Now that you have been introduced to a variety of herbal preparations and how to make them, all that's left to do is head to the kitchen and get started! If you're wondering where on earth you should begin, let me remind you once more to let the seasons guide you.

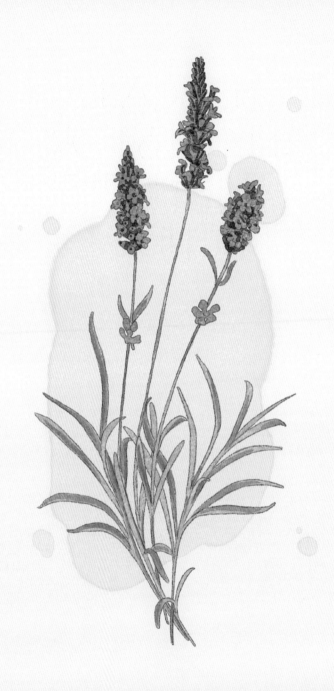

SEASONAL RECIPES FOR THE HOME APOTHECARY

Just as the natural world transforms around us each season, our bodies and minds also ebb and flow with the cycles of the year. By aligning ourselves with nature's rhythms and incorporating seasonal herbs into our daily lives, we can tap into the profound wisdom of seasonal herbalism and experience a harmonious connection with nature.

The following pages contain a collection of carefully curated herbal recipes intended to support your health and wellness throughout each season of the year.

During the vibrancy of spring, explore herbal oils, ointments, and washes that soothe and protect the skin as you venture outdoors once more. In the radiant heat of summer, indulge in refreshing herbal infusions and cooling muscle oils to help you beat the heat and promote vitality. As autumn paints the world in shades of muted colors, uncover recipes for immune-boosting herbal syrups and warming herbal broths to help you transition from one season to the next with grace and resilience. And when winter's chill descends, cozy up with recipes for soothing herbal balms, respiratory steams, and infused honeys that fortify the body's defenses and offer you solace during the cold months.

Whether you are an experienced herbalist or a curious newcomer to the wild and wonderful world of herbs, these herbal recipes will inspire and empower you on your journey to becoming a seasonal herbalist. Each recipe combines the wisdom of traditional herbalism with a touch of creativity, inviting you to embark on your own herbal adventures and forge a deeper connection with the power of plants and the seasons that guide us all.

But first—a couple of things before you head off to the kitchen to begin making your seasonal preparations.

The herbal recipes that follow generally call for dry plant material unless fresh plant material is specifically mentioned. However, if you want to use fresh plant material instead of dried, you will need to double the volume measurement (not weight) of the herb called for in the recipe to account for the extra water content in the fresh plant material.

For example, if a recipe calls for 2 tablespoons (4 grams) peppermint (*Mentha* x *piperita*) leaf, and you want to use fresh peppermint, you will need to use 4 tablespoons, which should still come to approximately 4 grams of weight instead.

Most of the recipes in this book can be easily doubled or tripled to create larger batches or cut in half to create smaller batches depending on your preferences and use of the recipe. I recommend you make the recipe as written the first time. If you find yourself running out of it quickly, make a note to double the recipe the next time you make it. If you find yourself not using it before reaching its expiration date, make a note to reduce the recipe.

So, let us set off on this transformative journey as we embrace the magic of the seasons and unlock the secrets of nature's herbal bounty. Welcome to the realm of seasonal herbal recipes for the home apothecary, where wellness and nourishment await at every turn.

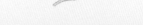

SPRING

Spring is one of my favorite seasons, both as an herbalist and a gardener. After the long, cold days of winter, the first sign of green plants emerging from the warming soil sets my heart aflutter and beckons me outdoors to explore the land for more signs of new life. As I dig my fingers in the thawing soil and breathe in its scent, I begin to plan the gardens and harvests to come. The potential of the season fills me with anticipation and hope in such a way that I'm caught off guard by it every year.

In spring, plenty of herbs are available for harvest. Bitter roots are accessible when the soil is soft enough to dig. The bark from trees and shrubs is ready to harvest when the sap starts running again. Leaves and tender aboveground plant parts are ready to gather all season long. Spring buds and flowers are free for the taking as soon as they make their appearance too!

Depending on your location and climate, some common herbs you might find during the spring season include:

- Aerial and aboveground parts: chickweed (*Stellaria media*), cleavers (*Galium aparine*), ground ivy (*Glechoma hederacea*), nettle (*Urtica dioica*), purple dead nettle (*Lamium purpureum*)

- Bark: birch (*Betula* spp.), crampbark (*Viburnum opulus*), oak (*Quercus* spp.), sassafras (*Sassafras albidum*), wild cherry (*Prunus serotina*), willow (*Salix* spp.), witch hazel (*Hamamelis virginiana*)

- Buds and flowers: coltsfoot (*Tussilago farfara*), dandelion (*Taraxacum officinale*), forsythia (*Forsythia suspensa*), poplar (*Populus* spp.), rose (*Rosa* spp.), violet (*Viola odorata*)

- Leaves: comfrey (*Symphytum officinale*), dandelion (*Taraxacum officinale*), mullein (*Verbascum thapsus*), plantain (*Plantago* spp.), yarrow (*Achillea millefolium*), violet (*Viola* spp.)

- Roots: burdock (*Arctium lappa*), dandelion (*Taraxacum officinale*), yellow dock (*Rumex crispus*)

Just as nature awakes from its winter slumber, we, too, must slowly emerge from a quiet, restful state as our energy levels rise gradually throughout the spring season. We can use this ever-increasing energy to help guide us to make healthy choices that benefit our wellness. One such choice is transitioning our diet away from the hardy foods of winter toward the lighter foods of spring, which may look like eating more wild edible greens as soon as they become available, either gently cooked or eaten raw. This is also the perfect time to introduce bitter flavors from roots and leaves into our diet, which help support the liver and digestive systems and set the body up to break down and absorb important nutrients. It's also important to make sure we're getting plenty of healthy fats and staying hydrated with mineral-rich fluids as increasing temperatures and activity levels throughout the season can lead to dry tissues.

As we transition from winter to spring, we also find that ailments and seasonal conditions begin to shift away from those common in winter toward those more common in spring. Plants and trees begin to bloom, insects buzz about, and the weather grows steadily warmer. Depending on location, there might be a lot of humidity in the air due to increased rainfall. We often spend more time outdoors, and it's not uncommon to find ourselves dealing with a variety of respiratory issues, skin irritations, digestive upsets, and other troubles associated with the seasonal adjustments of spring.

Here, you will find botanical recipes that can come to your aid when potential ailments and seasonal conditions come your way during the spring season.

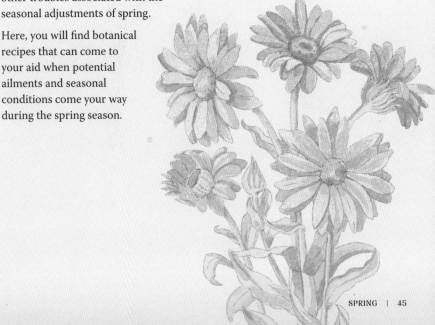

Spring Reset Chai Tea

Give the body a gentle (and tasty) wake-up with liver-supportive herbs and circulatory stimulating spices that will encourage healthy energy flow and metabolic function—the perfect daily sipper to help you transition from winter to spring.

YIELD: 2 CUPS (480 ML)

Ingredients

2 cups (480 mL) water

2-3 tbsp (14–21 g) Spring Reset Chai tea blend (below)

1 cup (240 mL) milk

Raw honey, to taste (optional)

Spring Reset Chai Tea Blend:

2 parts dandelion (*Taraxacum officinale*) root

1 part chicory (*Cichorium intybus*) root

1 part cinnamon (*Cinnamomum verum*) bark

½ part clove (*Syzygium aromaticum*) bud

½ part cardamom *Elettaria cardamomum*) pods, crushed

½ part black pepper (*Piper nigrum*) seeds

½ part ginger (*Zingiber officinale*) rhizome

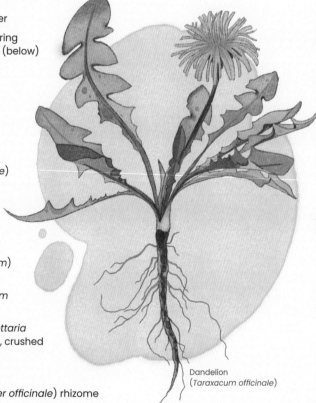

Dandelion
(*Taraxacum officinale*)

Directions

1 Start by blending your Spring Reset Chai tea blend together. Measure out each herb individually and combine them in a large mixing bowl, stirring the herbs well to fully blend them together. Transfer this tea blend to a labeled glass storage container. Cap and store for future use.

2 Place 2–3 tbsp (14-21 g) of Spring Reset Chai tea blend in a small saucepan. Pour 2 cups (480 mL) of water over the plant material, stirring the mixture well to fully saturate the herbs with water, and place a lid on the saucepan. Allow this mixture to sit for 12–24 hours, giving the harder plant parts time to soften, if desired.

3 When you are ready to make the tea, place the saucepan on the stove, remove the lid, and bring the mixture to a boil over medium-high heat. When the water comes to a boil, immediately reduce the heat to bring the mixture to a simmer. Add 1 cup (240 mL) milk and hold the mixture at a simmer until the liquid has reduced to 2 cups (480 mL).

4 Once the liquid has reduced to 2 cups (480 mL), carefully strain the mixture through a fine-mesh sieve (lined with a few layers of cheesecloth to remove any plant material, if you wish). Press the herbs with the back of a spoon (or gather the edges of the cheesecloth to create a bundle and squeeze) to extract as much liquid as possible. Reserve the liquid in a clean, heat-proof mug or glass canning jar and compost the used plant material. Sweeten with raw honey, if desired.

Usage

Drink up to 2 cups (480 mL) a day, hot or cold.

Storage & Shelf-life

Store tea blend in a cool, dark location. Use within 12 months before making a fresh batch.

Spring Allergy–Ease Infusion

From pollinating trees and blooming flowers to mowing grass and harvesting hay—spring allergy season can feel never-ending for those who suffer from seasonal allergies. Thankfully, you can access the inflammation-modulating and histamine-calming properties of fresh nettle through this refreshing herbal infusion all throughout the season.

YIELD: 4 CUPS (960 ML)

Ingredients

4 cups (960 mL) water

2 cups (28 g) fresh nettle (*Urtica dioica*) tops

2 tbsp (4 g) peppermint (*Mentha x piperita*) leaf for flavor (optional)

Local raw honey, to taste (optional)

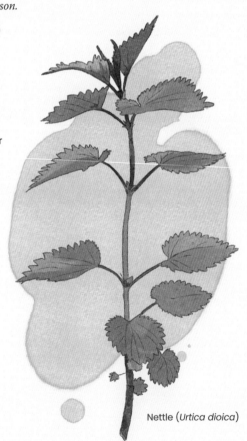

Nettle (*Urtica dioica*)

Directions

1 Wearing protective gloves, cut the top 4–6 inches from each nettle plant. This will encourage the plant to produce more leaves, ensuring plenty of nettles all season. Carefully rinse the nettle leaves under cool running water to wash away debris, and thoroughly shake them to remove excess water.

2 When you are ready to make your infusion, bring 4 cups (960 mL) of water to a boil in a kettle or a small saucepan over medium-high heat. As soon as the water comes to a boil, remove it from the heat.

3 While the water is coming to a boil, roughly chop the nettle wearing protective gloves. Weigh out 28 g of nettle (approximately 2 cups) on a kitchen scale, and transfer the leaves to a clean glass canning jar. Feel free to add 2 tbsp (4 g) peppermint, or another flavorful herb, to adjust the flavor to your preference. It can also help improve the flavor to serve it over ice.

4 Pour 4 cups (960 mL) of boiled water over the ingredients, cap, and set aside to infuse up to 4 hours (or overnight for a long-steep infusion).

5 When time is up, carefully strain the mixture through a fine-mesh sieve (lined with a few layers of cheesecloth to remove any plant material, if you wish). Press the herbs with the back of a spoon (or gather the edges of the cheesecloth to create a bundle and squeeze) to extract as much liquid as possible. Reserve the liquid in a clean glass storage container and compost the used plant material.

6 Sweeten with local raw honey, if desired. Cap and store for future use.

To support allergies, fresh nettle is best, as the drying process reduces the plant constituents that lend themselves to easing inflammation and the histamine response. Nettle can be grown from seed, foraged in the wild, or even purchased from local farmer's markets. If fresh nettle isn't available to you, or you aren't a fan of herbal infusions, freeze-dried nettle capsules also contain all the beneficial phytochemicals you need. These are best taken 2–4 weeks before allergy season begins and throughout the season for maximum results.

Substitute fresh goldenrod (*Solidago* spp.) aerial parts in place of the nettle in the autumn for an equally helpful infusion for autumn allergies!

Usage

Drink 4 cups (960 mL) of nettle infusion, hot or cold, daily throughout allergy season.

Storage & Shelf-life

Store the prepared infusion in the refrigerator for no more than 24 hours before making a fresh batch.

Tips

- While it's best to use freshly harvested nettle right away, you can wrap them in a damp towel and store them in the refrigerator for 24–48 hours.
- Reserve the used nettle leaf from your infusion to include in an upcoming recipe (freeze them if you don't plan to use them in a day or so) or compost them to amend your soil (adding nutrients to the soil).
- If you don't want to make this infusion on a daily basis, feel free to triple or quadruple the batch and freeze the extra liquid, thawing it the night before you need it.

Sinus Soother Rinse

This must-have herbal sinus rinse is a great way to gently cleanse nasal and sinus passages of irritants and debris while moisturizing dry tissues and helping you to breathe a bit easier this spring.

YIELD: 4 CUPS (960 ML)

Ingredients

¼ cup (16 g) olive (*Olea europaea*) leaf

3 tbsp (10 g) eucalyptus (*Eucalyptus globulus*) leaf

2 tbsp (3 g) violet (*Viola odorata*) leaf

1 tbsp (2 g) plantain (*Plangato* spp.) leaf

1 tbsp (1 g) rose (*Rosa* spp.) petal

1 tbsp (18 g) baking soda

4 cups (960 mL) water

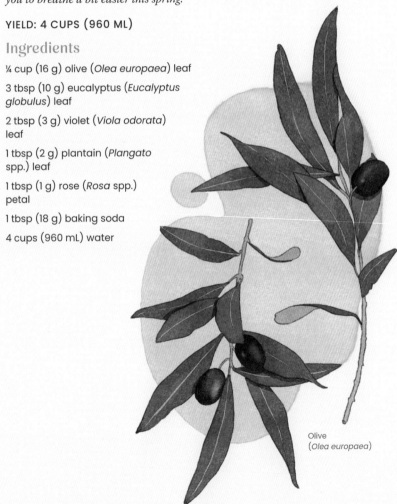

Olive
(*Olea europaea*)

Directions

1 Bring 4 cups (960 mL) of water to a boil in a kettle or a small saucepan over medium-high heat. As soon as the water comes to a boil, remove it from the heat.

2 While the water is coming to a boil, combine herbs and baking soda together in a quart-sized glass canning jar.

3 Pour 4 cups (960 mL) of boiled water over the ingredients, cap, and set aside to infuse for 20 minutes or up to 4 hours (or overnight for a long-steep infusion).

4 When time is up, carefully strain the mixture through a fine-mesh sieve lined with an unbleached coffee filter to remove any fine particles (you don't want bits of herbs in your sinus cavities!). Press the herbs with the back of a spoon (or gather the edges of the coffee filter to create a bundle and gently squeeze) to extract as much liquid as possible. Reserve the liquid in a clean glass storage container and compost the used plant material. Cap and store for future use.

Usage

Add 1 cup (240 mL) of warm liquid to a neti pot or nasal irrigation bottle. Use as directed to rinse the nasal and sinus passages 3–4 times a day.

Storage & Shelf-life

Store extras in the refrigerator for no more than 24 hours before making a fresh batch.

Tip

• You can reuse strained herbs 1–2 more times before composting them (just add more baking soda for each repeated infusion). While subsequent infusions will be slightly weaker than the first, they will still extract plant constituents that remain in the plant material and will be beneficial to the sinus tissues.

LUNG LOVE SYRUP

Show your lungs some love with this tasty syrup that is not only toning to the tissues—providing strength and support for proper function—but also eases inflammation, thins thick mucus, and soothes irritation all at the same time. Whether you have prevention or recovery in mind, this syrup will come to your aid.

YIELD: 4 CUPS (960 ML)

Ingredients

6 tbsp (8 g) mullein (*Verbascum thapsus*) leaf

6 tbsp (12 g) plantain (*Plantago* spp.) leaf

6 tbsp (5 g) goldenrod (*Solidago* spp.) aerial parts

4 tbsp (8 g) tulsi (*Ocimum tenuiflorum*) aerial parts

2 tbsp (16 g) elecampane (*Inula helenium*) root

2 tbsp (10 g) astragalus (*Astragalus mongholicus*) root

2 tbsp (4 g) peppermint (*Mentha x piperita*) leaf

4 cups (960 mL) water

2 cups (480 mL) raw honey

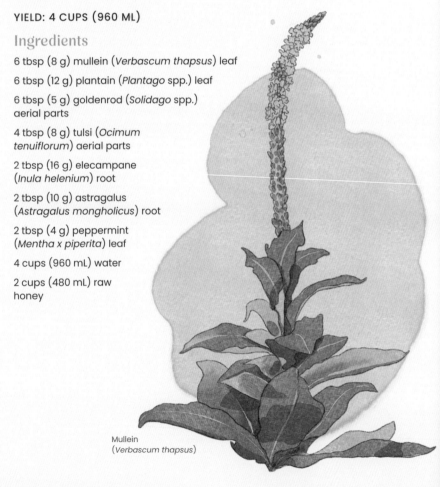

Mullein
(*Verbascum thapsus*)

Directions

1 Measure all herbs, except for peppermint, and combine them together in a small saucepan. Pour 4 cups (960 mL) of water over the plant material, stirring the mixture well to fully saturate the herbs with water, and place a lid on the saucepan. Allow this mixture to sit for 12–24 hours, giving the harder plant parts time to soften, if desired.

2 When you are ready to make the syrup, place the saucepan on the stove, remove the lid, and bring the mixture to a boil over medium-high heat. When the water comes to a boil, immediately reduce the heat to bring the mixture to a simmer and hold it there until the water level has reduced by half—to 2 cups (480 mL)—to create a decoction.

3 Once the water level has reduced to 2 cups (480 mL), remove the saucepan from the heat and add the peppermint leaf to the mixture, being sure to submerge it into the hot liquid. Immediately cover the saucepan with a lid, and allow the mixture to steep for 20 minutes.

4 When time is up, carefully strain the decoction through a fine-mesh sieve (lined with a few layers of cheesecloth to remove any plant material, if you wish). Press the herbs with the back of a spoon (or gather the edges of the cheesecloth to create a bundle and squeeze) to extract as much liquid as possible. Reserve the decocted liquid in a clean glass measuring cup, adding more water, if needed, to bring the total volume of liquid up to 2 cups (480 mL), and compost the used plant material.

5 Allow the liquid to cool slightly before adding 2 cups (480 mL) of raw honey. Stir well to combine and transfer to a labeled glass storage container. Cap and store for future use.

Usage

Use 1 tbsp (15 mL) of syrup 3 times a day for 4–6 weeks. Take straight off the spoon, mix with some seltzer water, or add to a smoothie or yogurt bowl.

Storage & Shelf-life

Store syrup in the refrigerator. Use within 3–4 weeks before making a fresh batch.

Botanical Bug Spray

Deter pesky bugs (and their bites) with the help of aromatic botanicals! Simply spritz this bug-repellent spray onto your clothes as often as needed to stay bug-free as you head outdoors this spring.

YIELD: ½ CUP (120 ML)

Ingredients

½ cup (120 mL) yarrow (*Achillea millefolium*) hydrosol

2 tsp (10 mL) of thick aloe (*Aloe vera*) gel

25 drops of lavender (*Lavendula angustifolia*) essential oil

15 drops of geranium (*Pelargonium graveolens*) essential oil

8 drops of patchouli (*Pogostemom cablin*) essential oil

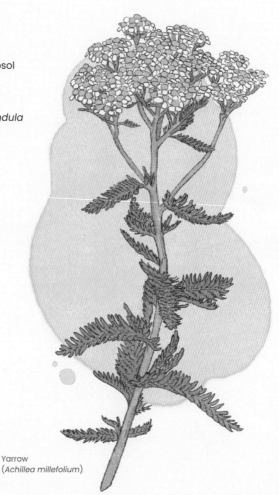

Yarrow
(*Achillea millefolium*)

Directions

1 Measure and combine all ingredients in a bowl to create a 2% dilution, which is the suggested dilution for use in products that cover a larger surface area of the body.

2 Blend the mixture using an immersion blender or personal blender until all ingredients are well incorporated.

3 Transfer the mixture to a labeled glass bottle and cap with a spray top. Store for future use.

Usage

Shake well before using to ensure ingredients are combined. Lightly spritz the mixture over clothes before heading outdoors, doing your best to avoid the skin. Reapply as often as needed to keep bugs at bay.

Storage & Shelf-life

Store in a cool, dark location. Use within one month before making a fresh batch.

Tip

• Add these essential oils to ½ cup (120 mL) of a carrier oil of your choice to create a bug-deterring body oil that you can apply to your skin.

Yarrow is a must-have herb in any herbal garden because of its wide array of uses. Grow it from seed, purchase it at a local nursery (be sure you're getting an organic heirloom variety instead of a hybrid for best results), or harvest it from the wild after proper identification (as it has some poisonous look-alikes!). Yarrow's beneficial properties are primarily attributed to its volatile oil content, which is also responsible for its strong aroma.

INSECT STING POULTICE

Just as we come out of our time of winter rest, so do the insects. The pain from bees, wasps, and other insect stings can be, well, quite painful. Thankfully, there is an herb that grows far and wide all over the world and is known for its usefulness in easing the uncomfortable symptoms of these types of stings. Plantain leaf is an herb that not only helps to ease pain and swelling but soothes tissues and stimulates quicker cell regeneration as well.

YIELD: VARIES

Ingredients

2–3 fresh plantain (*Plantago* spp.) leaves, chopped

1–2 tbsp (15–30 mL) cool water

Directions

1 Place fresh plantain leaf in a personal blender and add 1 tbsp (15 mL) of water. Blend until the herb becomes a pulp, adding more water, if needed.

2 Strain the mixture through a fine-mesh sieve, reserving the pulp and liquid separately.

Usage

Place a small amount of plantain pulp directly on the sting site (after carefully removing the stinger if stung by a honey bee) and cover it with a clean bandage. Leave this poultice on for 2–3 hours. Apply more of the reserved pulp if pain and swelling are still present and rebandage. Drink the reserved liquid from step 2 to further ease inflammation and slow histamine release in the body. Feel free to drink the liquid straight, dilute it in a small amount of water, or mix it into a smoothie.

Storage & Shelf-life

Reserve extra pulp in a clean glass container in the refrigerator and use it within 24 hours before making a fresh batch.

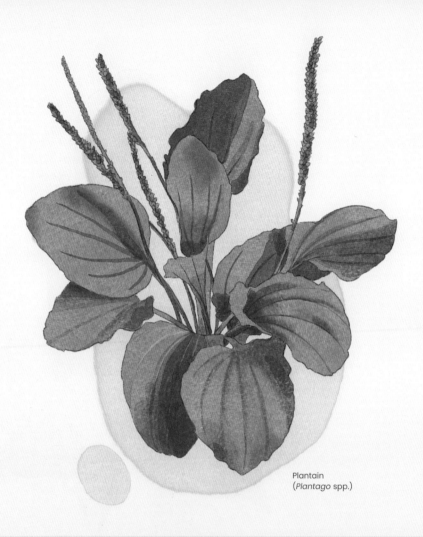

Plantain
(*Plantago* spp.)

If you are stung outdoors and don't have access to a blender, you can simply wipe a couple of fresh plantain leaves clean of dirt and debris on your shirt (or rinse them in a nearby clean water source), pop them into your mouth, chew away, spit the pulp out, and put the chewed leaves directly on your sting. This is called a "spit poultice," and it's a traditional way to make a poultice when you don't have the convenience of electricity!

ITCH–EASE HERBAL OIL

Itchy bug bites (and rashes) are the worst. Thankfully, we have some great herbal allies that can come to our aid when itchy things ail us. This herb-infused oil is a simple way to ease the itch and soothe minor swelling and irritation that often accompany bug bites.

YIELD: ¼–½ CUP (60–120 ML)

Ingredients

¼–½ cup (60-120 mL) olive oil

1 tbsp (6 g) clove (*Syzygium aromaticum*) bud

1 tbsp (2 g) plantain (*Plantago* spp.) leaf

1 tbsp (1 g) calendula (*Calendula officinalis*) flower

2 tsp (1 g) violet (*Viola odorata*) leaf

60-120 drops of peppermint (*Mentha* x *piperita*) essential oil (or lavender (*Lavandula angustifolia*) essential oil for children <6 years old)

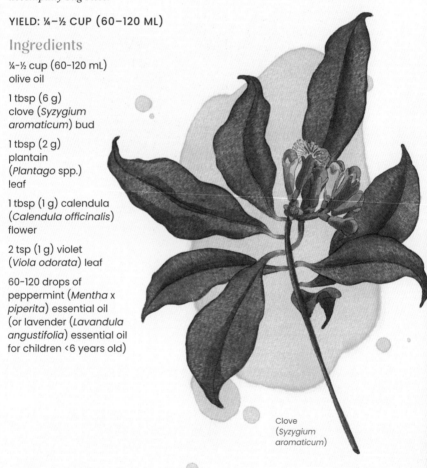

Clove
(*Syzygium aromaticum*)

Directions

1 Measure all ingredients and follow the steps for the quick or slow herb-infused oil method on pages 32–34.

2 When your oil is finished, place a fine-mesh sieve (lined with a few layers of cheesecloth to remove plant material, if you wish) over a clean, dry glass container and carefully pour the mixture through it. Press the herbs with the back of a spoon (or gather the edges of the cheesecloth to create a bundle and gently squeeze) to extract as much liquid as possible. You can double strain the decanted liquid once more through a fine-mesh sieve lined with an unbleached coffee filter to further remove fine particles if you wish and compost the used plant material.

3 Use a glass measuring cup or graduated cylinder to measure the amount of herb-infused oil you have. If needed, add more olive oil to bring the total volume of oil back up to the amount you started with: ¼–½ cup (60–120 mL).

4 Add 60 drops of essential oil for every ¼ cup (60 mL) of herb-infused oil to create a 5% dilution, which is the suggested dilution for use on small surface areas of the body during acute issues.

5 Mix well with a spoon. Transfer the finished oil to labeled glass roller bottles and allow it to cool completely. Once cool, cap and store for future use.

Usage

Roll a small amount of oil directly onto itchy bug bites or rashes as often as needed. Discontinue use if irritation occurs.

Storage & Shelf-life

Store in a cool, dark location. Use within 12 months before making a fresh batch.

Clove contains a compound called eugenol, which is primarily responsible for its temporary numbing effect on the skin. When applied to the skin, eugenol interacts with nerve endings, blocking the transmission of pain signals to the brain. This is why clove oil or other clove-based products are often used topically to ease pain. However, it's essential to use clove oil or products containing clove with caution, as excessive application can lead to skin irritation or other adverse reactions.

HERBAL EYEWASH

As the days warm, a variety of eye irritants can be problematic for us as we open the windows to let the fresh spring air in and begin to spend more time outdoors. Whether you have an irritant in your eye or the eye is red, painful, and swollen, this herbal eyewash can help rinse and soothe the delicate tissues of the eye thanks to the bacterial-suppressing, inflammation-modulating, and emollient properties of the botanicals in this blend.

YIELD: 8 FL OZ (240 ML)

Ingredients

1 cup (240 mL) water

3 tbsp (5 g) chamomile
(*Matricaria chamomilla*)
flower

3 tbsp (3 g) calendula
(*Calendula officinalis*)
flower

2 tbsp (4 g) yarrow
(*Achillea millefolium*)
aerial parts

2 tbsp (3 g) violet
(*Viola* spp.) leaf

½ tsp (4 g) sea salt

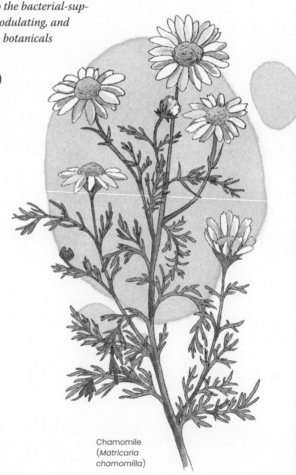

Chamomile
(*Matricaria
chamomilla*)

Directions

1 Bring 1 cup (240 mL) of water to a boil in a kettle or a small saucepan over medium-high heat. As soon as the water comes to a boil, remove it from the heat.

2 While the water is coming to a boil, combine herbs and salt together in a pint-sized glass canning jar.

3 Pour 1 cup (240 mL) of boiled water over the ingredients, cap, and set the jar aside to infuse for 20 minutes or up to 4 hours (or overnight for a long-steep infusion).

4 When time is up, carefully strain the mixture through a fine-mesh sieve lined with an unbleached coffee filter to remove any fine particles (you don't want bits of herbs in your eyes!). Press the herbs with the back of a spoon (or gather the edges of the coffee filter to create a bundle and gently squeeze) to extract as much liquid as possible. Reserve the liquid in a clean glass storage container and compost the used plant material. Cap and store for future use.

Usage

To use as an eye wash, fill an eye wash cup half full with warm herbal eye wash. Holding your head over a sink, bring the cup up to your eye and hold it firmly to avoid leaks. Tilt your head back so that the liquid covers your eye. Blink a few times, moving the eyeball back and forth so the liquid covers the entire surface. Tilt your head back down and remove the eye cup. Rinse and dry the cup for storage, and gently dry the eye. Repeat 3–4 times a day.

To use as an eye compress, soak a clean cloth in the warm herbal eye wash and press out just enough liquid that it's not dripping from the cloth. Fold the wet cloth into a square and place it over the eye. Hold it firmly to the eye for 10 minutes. Repeat with a clean cloth 3–4 times a day.

Storage & Shelf-life

Store in a labeled jar in the refrigerator for no more than 24 hours before making a fresh batch.

Tip

• Feel free to double or triple the recipe if it will be used for several days. Freeze leftovers in ice cube trays and thaw them as needed, warming the liquid to a comfortable temperature before using.

All-Purpose Herbal Ointment

Spring has a way of drawing us outdoors, whether it's to pick the first wildflowers that bloom, go for a hike in the warming temperatures, or dig in the dirt to get a head start on the year's garden. This all-purpose herbal ointment is infused with herbs that deter microbes and stimulate tissue regeneration and will come in handy for minor cuts, scrapes, and abrasions that may come your way during your outdoor adventures.

YIELD: ½–1 CUP (120–240 ML)

Ingredients

½–1 cup (120-240 mL) olive oil

1 cup (14 g) calendula (*Calendula officinalis*) flower

¼ cup (7 g) lavender (*Lavandula* spp.) flower bud

¼ cup (5 g) yarrow (*Achillea millefolium*) aerial parts

2 tbsp (4 g) comfrey (*Symphytum officinale*) leaf

3–6 tbsp (21–42 g) beeswax, grated or pastille

60–120 drops of lavender (*Lavandula angustifolia*) essential oil (optional)

60–120 drops of tea tree (*Melaleuca alternifolia*) essential oil (optional)

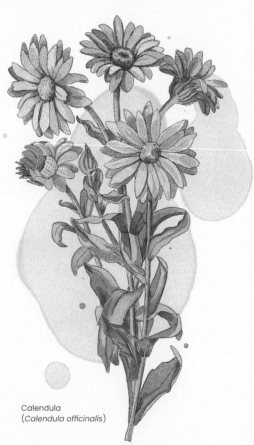

Calendula
(*Calendula officinalis*)

Directions

1 Measure all ingredients and follow the steps for the quick or slow herb-infused oil method on pages 32–34.

2 When your oil is finished, place a fine-mesh sieve (lined with a few layers of cheesecloth to remove plant material, if you wish) over a clean, dry glass container and carefully pour the mixture through it. Press the herbs with the back of a spoon (or gather the edges of the cheesecloth to create a bundle and gently squeeze) to extract as much liquid as possible. You can double strain the decanted liquid once more through a fine-mesh sieve lined with an unbleached coffee filter to further remove fine particles if you wish and compost the used plant material.

3 When you are ready to make the ointment, use a glass measuring cup or graduated cylinder to measure the amount of herb-infused oil you have. If needed, add more olive oil to bring the total volume of oil back up to the amount you started with: ½–1 cup (120–240 mL).

4 Measure out 3 tbsp (21 g) of beeswax for every ½ cup (120 mL) of herb-infused oil you have. Place the beeswax into a clean saucepan, and heat it over medium-low heat until it has melted.

5 Turn the heat to low and pour the herb-infused oil into the saucepan alongside the melted beeswax. Carefully mix the two together until they're thoroughly combined.

6 Test the consistency of the ointment by dipping a spoon in the mixture and letting it cool for a few minutes before touching it to get a feel for the final consistency. The goal is for the texture to be soft and easy to press. If the mixture is too hard, add a bit more oil. If the mixture is too soft, add another 1 tbsp (7 g) of beeswax. Be sure to go slow and make small adjustments, testing after each addition and repeating until you get the ointment to the desired consistency.

7 Remove the saucepan from the heat and carefully transfer the mixture to a labeled tin or glass storage container.

8 If using, add 60 drops of each essential oil for every ½ cup (120 mL) of herb-infused oil to create a 5% dilution, which is the suggested dilution for use on small surface areas of the body during acute injury. Stir the mixture with a toothpick and allow it to cool completely. Once cool, cap and store for future use.

Usage

With a clean finger, scoop a small amount of ointment out of the storage container. Apply directly to minor wounds and abrasions as often as needed.

Storage & Shelf-life

Store in a cool, dark location. Use within 12 months before making a fresh batch.

Calendula is one of the easiest herbs to grow! Sow seeds in a container or directly in the ground, cover them with a small amount of dirt, water well, and sit back and watch beautiful yellow-orange blooms appear in a couple of months. Calendula flowers should be picked as soon as they're in full bloom, stimulating the growth of more flowers and giving you a long harvest period. Calendula can be used fresh or dried for future use. Don't forget to let some of the flowers go to seed so you can collect the seeds and replant them the following year.

Herbal Earache Oil

Breezy spring days and temperature fluctuations, along with spring allergies and viral ailments, can sometimes lead to uncomfortable earaches. Thankfully, there are some tried-and-true herbal combinations that can quickly be infused in oil and used inside the ear canal to help ease pain and swelling and deter microbes.

YIELD: ¼–½ CUP (60–120 ML)

Ingredients

¼–½ cup (60-120 mL) olive oil

1 tbsp (1 g) mullein
(*Verbascum thapsus*) flower

1 tbsp (2 g) bee balm
(*Monarda fistulosa*) aerial parts

2 (12 g) garlic (*Allium sativum*)
cloves, minced

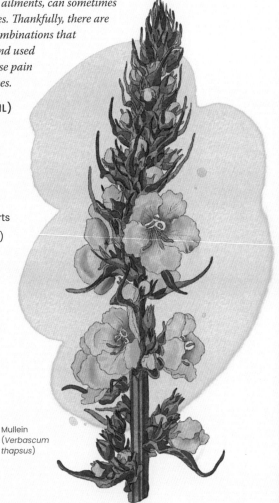

Mullein
(*Verbascum
thapsus*)

Directions

1 Measure all ingredients and follow the steps for the quick herb-infused oil method on pages 32–33.

2 When your oil is finished, place a fine-mesh sieve (lined with a few layers of cheesecloth to remove plant material, if you wish) over a clean, dry glass container and carefully pour the mixture through it. Press the herbs with the back of a spoon (or gather the edges of the cheesecloth to create a bundle and gently squeeze) to extract as much liquid as possible. You can double strain the decanted liquid once more through a fine-mesh sieve lined with an unbleached coffee filter to further remove fine particles if you wish and compost the used plant material.

3 Transfer the finished oil to a clean, labeled glass storage container and set aside to cool. Once cool, cap with a dropper top and store for future use.

Usage

Warm the oil by placing the bottle in a cup of hot water for 10–15 minutes. Apply 2–3 drops of oil into the canal of the affected ear, keeping the ear tilted upward for 5–10 minutes so the oil doesn't run back out. Repeat 2–3 times a day. You can also massage a small amount of this oil into the skin around the ear and down the neck, gently massaging to encourage lymphatic drainage and oil absorption.

Storage & Shelf-life

Store in a cool, dark location. Use within 12 months before making a fresh batch.

Garlic contains several phytochemicals, including allicin and other sulfur compounds, that contribute to its antiviral and antibacterial action. These make it an effective herbal ally against a wide spectrum of bacteria, including many strains of antibiotic-resistant bacteria.

Aromatic Earache Oil

Essential oils not only smell nice, but they're also useful resources to have on hand during an earache. They help relax tension, ease inflammation, and calm the nerves, and they can discourage microbial growth as well.

YIELD: ¼ CUP (60 ML)

Ingredients

¼ cup (60 mL) olive oil

16–24 drops of tea tree (*Melaleuca alternifolia*) essential oil

12–20 drops of basil (*Ocimum basilicum*) essential oil

8–16 drops of lavender (*Lavandula angustifolia*) essential oil

Directions

1 Combine olive oil (or another herb-infused oil of your choice) and essential oils together to create a 3–5% dilution, which is the suggested dilution for use on small surface areas of the body during acute issues.

2 Transfer the finished oil to a clean, labeled glass storage container and cap. Shake well to thoroughly mix the oils together and store for future use.

Usage

Apply a small amount of oil to the skin around the ear and down the neck, gently massaging to encourage lymphatic drainage and oil absorption. Reapply 3–4 times a day. For external use only!

Storage & Shelf-life

Store in a cool, dark location. Use within 12 months before making a fresh batch.

Tip

• This oil can also discourage microbial growth and inflammation in other areas of the skin. It makes a great preparation to rub on cleaned cuts, scrapes, and scratches.

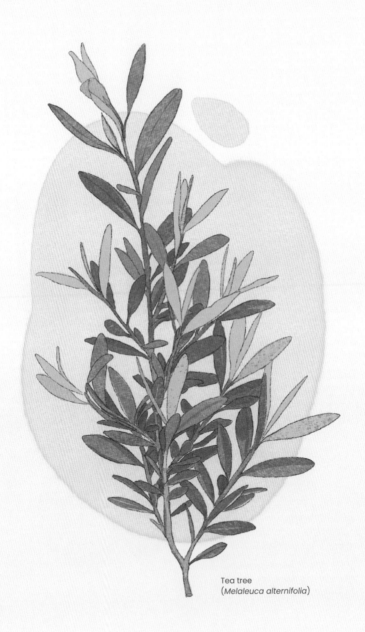

Tea tree
(*Melaleuca alternifolia*)

Black Drawing Salve

With the arrival of spring, you will likely find yourself spending more time out-doors. Black drawing salve is a traditional Amish preparation that has stood the test of time thanks to its effectiveness in drawing impurities from the skin's surface, such as splinters, thorns, small gravel, and dirt. It's also commonly used on venomous insect bites and boils to help slow venom spread and draw toxins and impurities out of the skin.

YIELD: ¾ CUP (180 ML)

Ingredients

2 tbsp (14 g) beeswax, grated or pastille

3 tbsp (45 mL) olive oil

1 tbsp (15 mL) castor oil

2 tbsp (24 g) activated charcoal

2 tbsp (20 g) bentonite clay

1 tbsp (2 g) plantain (*Plantago* spp.) leaf, powdered

1 tbsp (15 mL) raw honey

¼ tsp (1 mL) vitamin E oil (optional)

28 drops of lavender (*Lavandula angustifolia*) essential oil (optional)

8 drops of tea tree (*Melaleuca alternifolia*) essential oil (optional)

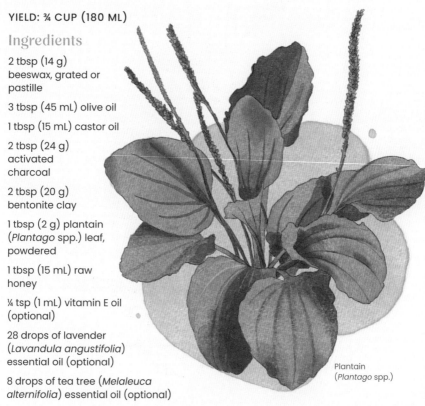

Plantain
(*Plantago* spp.)

Directions

1 Measure out 2 tbsp (14 g) of beeswax. Place it into a clean saucepan and heat it over medium-low heat until it has melted.

2 Turn the heat to low and add the olive and castor oils to the saucepan alongside the melted beeswax. Carefully mix them together until they're thoroughly combined.

3 Remove the saucepan from heat and add the charcoal, clay, and plantain powders. Mix the powders into the oils before adding the raw honey and vitamin E oil, if using. Stir the mixture once more to incorporate all the ingredients together. Feel free to add extra clay or charcoal if you'd like a thicker consistency.

4 If using, add the essential oils to the mixture to create a 3% dilution, which is the suggested dilution for use on small surface areas of the body.

5 Transfer the mixture to a labeled glass storage container or tin and allow it to cool completely. Once cool, cap and store for future use.

Usage

Apply a small amount of clay to the affected area. Cover with a bandage and replace every 12 hours as needed.

Storage & Shelf-life

Store in a cool, dark location. Use within 12 months before making a fresh batch.

Tip

• You can create your own plantain leaf powder by placing 2–3 tbsp of dried plantain leaf in a coffee grinder and grinding it into a powder. Sift the powder through a fine-mesh sieve, reserving the fine powder and composting the larger particles. This creates quite a bit of dust, so be sure to do this in a well-ventilated area or wear a face mask.

The negative electrical charge of clay attracts the positive electrical charge of metal, binding the metal molecules to the clay and, depending on the type of clay, can sometimes render the clay less absorbent. For this reason, it is important to use non-reactive supplies, such as glass, enamel, or wood, when working with pure clay to ensure it is most effective.

Sore Throat Spray

If you find yourself with a dry, scratchy throat come spring, brought on by the cool, dry outdoor air, seasonal allergies, or an unexpected virus, this herbal throat spray is one of the best ways to soothe the painful tissues of the throat while combating microbes. Not only that, but it tastes great too!

YIELD: ½ CUP (120 ML)

Ingredients

2 tbsp (30 mL) raw honey

2 tbsp (30 mL) sage (*Salvia officinalis*) leaf tincture

2 tbsp (30 mL) licorice (*Glycyrrhiza glabra*) root tincture

2 tbsp (30 mL) echinacea (*Echinacea angustifolia, E. purpurea*) root tincture**

3–5 drops of eucalyptus (*Eucalyptus globulus*) essential oil (optional)

** cultivated source

Directions

1 Measure and combine all ingredients in a labeled glass bottle and cap with a spray top.

2 Shake well to combine and store for future use.

Usage

Shake well before each use. Use 2–3 sprays in the mouth, swishing the liquid around for several seconds before swallowing it slowly so it comes into as much contact with the tissues at the back of the throat as possible. Repeat as often as needed.

Storage & Shelf-life

Store in a cool, dark location. Use within 2 years before making a fresh batch.

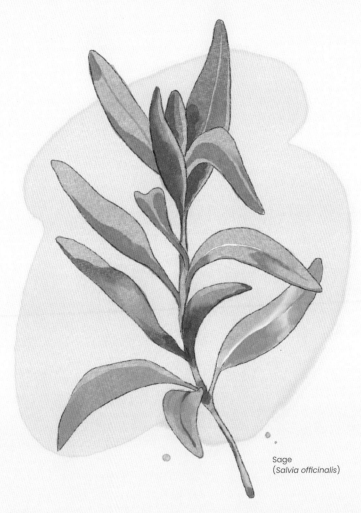

Sage
(*Salvia officinalis*)

Tips

- Need a safer essential oil for a younger child? No problem! Use fir needle (*Abies sibirica*) essential oil instead.

- If you have high blood pressure or kidney disease, skip the licorice root tincture and use fennel (*Foeniculum vulgare*) seed tincture instead.

Spring Digestive Bitters

If you're a seasonal eater, it's likely that you are shifting away from the heavier, richer fare of winter and toward the lighter, fresher fare of spring. This transition can sometimes be a challenge for the digestive system as it has to get used to a larger amount of fiber and raw foods once more. This transition can sometimes lead to slow digestion, bloating, gas, and even cramping. Thankfully, there are some herbs that can help support digestion and ease uncomfortable symptoms during this transition period—bitters! Bitter herbs stimulate gastric secretions and support digestion (among many other things). Plus, bitters infuse for less time than most tinctures since bitter principles are extracted from the plant material more quickly than other plant constituents.

YIELD: VARIES

Ingredients

3 parts dandelion (*Taraxacum officinale*) root tincture

2 parts chamomile (*Matricaria chamomilla*) flower tincture

2 parts cinnamon (*Cinnamomum* spp.) bark tincture

1 part yarrow (*Achillea millefolium*) aerial parts tincture

1 part orange (*Citrus* spp.) peel tincture

½ part fennel (*Foeniculum vulgare*) seed tincture

Directions

1 Make individual tinctures following directions on pages 35–38.

2 When you are ready to create the tincture blend, begin by choosing the measurement you'd like to use for your part.

3 Measure out each tincture individually before combining them in a clean, labeled glass storage container. Cap and store for future use.

Usage

Take ¼ tsp (1 mL) directly in the mouth 15–30 minutes before meals. Swish bitters over the tongue to taste the bitterness and stimulate salivation.

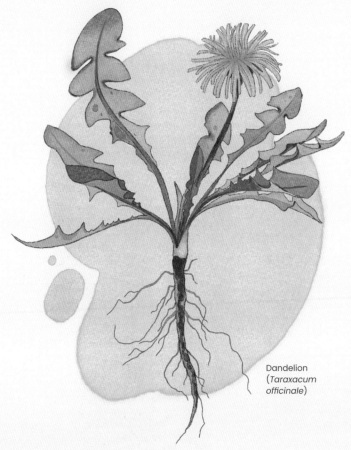

Dandelion
(*Taraxacum officinale*)

Storage & Shelf-life

Store in a cool, dark location. Use within 3–5 years before making a fresh batch.

Tips

- To make non-alcoholic spring digestive bitters, simply substitute raw apple cider vinegar for the alcohol when making each tincture. Use within 3 years.

- You can also use your bitters in your botanical cocktail and mocktail recipes.

- Place digestive bitters in a small, labeled spray bottle and keep it in your purse so you can take it with you on the go!

Lymph Love Succus

Spring is the ideal time to show the lymphatic system some love, especially after a long winter with less-than-average movement and a diet filled with heavy, seasonal foods. Come spring, there are some fresh green herbs that help to get the water pathways of the lymphatic system moving, which help to cleanse and refresh the body's tissues so they function better and give you renewed energy.

YIELD: VARIES

Ingredients

1 part fresh cleavers (*Galium aparine*) aboveground parts

1 part fresh chickweed (*Stellaria media*) aboveground parts

1 part fresh violet (*Viola* spp.) leaf

Water (optional)

70% ABV (or higher) alcohol of your choice

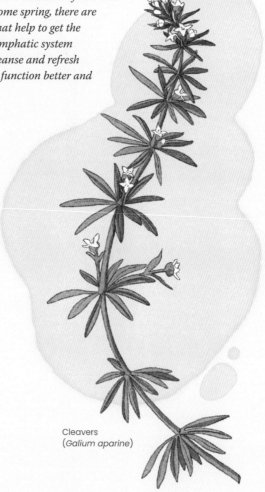

Cleavers
(*Galium aparine*)

Directions

1 Wearing protective gloves, collect the aboveground parts of fresh cleavers and chickweed, as well as violet leaf. Rinse the plants under cool running water to wash away debris, and thoroughly shake them to remove excess water.

2 Roughly chop the plant material before measuring each herb using your chosen part. Then, place the measured plant material in a large bowl.

3 To make a succus, you have two options.

   a First, you can process the fresh herbs with a juicer, reserving the juice in a clean glass storage container and composting the plant pulp.

   b If you don't have access to a juicer, you can combine the fresh plant material and a small amount of water in a high-speed blender and blend until a slurry forms, gradually adding more plant material (and additional water, if needed) until the mixture is well blended. Once the mixture is blended, strain it through a fine-mesh sieve lined with a few layers of cheesecloth to remove as much pulp as possible. Bundle the cheesecloth and squeeze as much liquid as possible from the plant material. Reserve the liquid in a clean glass storage container, and compost the used herbs.

4 Measure the amount of reserved liquid in a glass measuring cup or graduated cylinder and add an equal amount of 70% ABV (or higher) alcohol to preserve the liquid. For example, if you have 2 cups (480 mL) of liquid, you will need to add 2 cups (480 mL) of alcohol.

5 Transfer the mixture to a labeled glass storage container. Cap and store for future use.

Usage

Use 1–3 tsp (5–15 mL) 3 times a day. Drink it straight from the spoon, mix it into a smoothie, or add it to an herbal infusion.

Storage & Shelf-life

Store in a cool, dark location. Use within 3 years before making a fresh batch.

Tips

- Want to go alcohol-free? Skip the high-proof alcohol and use food-grade vegetable glycerin instead. The shelf-life will decrease to 1 year before a fresh batch is needed. You'll want to aim for a 2:3 ratio of liquid to glycerin. For example, if you have 2 cups (480 mL) of liquid, you will need to add 3 cups (720 mL) of glycerin.

- Skip the alcohol and glycerin and freeze the succus in ice cube trays to enjoy later. The shelf-life will decrease to 6 months before a fresh batch is needed.

Cleavers, chickweed, and violet all grow in similar habitats in spring—moist, shady spots—so if you see one plant, look around, as the others are likely growing nearby. These plants like to stay cool, and cleavers and chickweed are best used fresh for maximum potency.

SUMMER

Ah, summer! A season when nature is at its peak, and I feel as if I am too. I delight in seeing so many colorful flowers emerge across the landscape, and watching the bees and butterflies visit as many as they can. Nature's abundance is at its height, and I find myself in my busiest season. There are so many plants to gather, process, and prepare that by the end of the season, I reward myself with a much needed vacation for the season's labor. Summer inspires me to work with plants more than any other season, whether it's stocking up on foundational herbal preparations for my home apothecary, brushing up on my plant identification and foraging skills, or diving deep into studying a handful of new soon-to-be herbal allies. There's just so much to do, see, and learn in this busy season!

In summer, the harvest is bountiful. While the leaves of many plants are continually harvested throughout the season, gathering the aerial and aboveground parts of plants takes priority during summer, particularly where aromatic plants are concerned, as their flowers contain the precious volatile oils that give these plants much of their beneficial properties. Berries and some seeds begin to appear in the later half of this season as well!

Depending on your location and climate, some common herbs you might find during the summer season include:

- Aerial and aboveground parts: anise hyssop (*Agastache foeniculum*), blue vervain (*Verbena hastata*), boneset (*Eupatorium perfoliatum*), borage (*Borago officinalis*), California poppy (*Escholschzia californica*), echinacea* (*Echinacea* spp.), goldenrod (*Solidago* spp.), jewelweed (*Impatiens capensis, I. pallida*), lady's mantle (*Alchemilla vulgaris*), lavender (*Lavandula* spp.), linden (*Tilia* spp.), meadowsweet (*Filipendula ulmaria*), mints (*Mentha* spp.), motherwort (*Leonurus cardiaca*), mugwort (*Artemisia vulgaris*), red clover (*Trifolium pratense*), self-heal (*Prunella vulgaris*), skullcap (*Scutellaria lateriflora*), spilanthes (*Acmella oleracea*), thyme (*Thymus vulgaris*), tulsi (*Ocimum tenuiflorum*), wild lettuce (*Lactuca virosa*), yarrow (*Achillea millefolium*)

- Berries: elder (*Sambucus nigra, S. canadensis*), hawthorn (*Crataegus* spp.), sumac (*Rhus* spp.)

- Flowers: bee balm (*Monarda fistulosa*), calendula (*Calendula officinalis*), chamomile (*Matricaria chamomilla*), cornsilk (*Zea mays*), elder (*Sambucus nigra, S. canadensis*), feverfew (*Tanacetum parthenium*), hawthorn (*Crataegus* spp.), hops (*Humulus lupulus*), mullein (*Verbascum thapsus*), rose (*Rosa* spp.), St. John's wort (*Hypericum perforatum*), wormwood (*Artemisia absinthium*)

- Leaf: hawthorn (*Crataegus* spp.), lemon balm (*Melissa officinalis*), oregano (*Origanum vulgare*), raspberry (*Rubus* spp.), sage (*Salvia officinalis*)

- Seeds: black walnut (*Juglans nigra*) hull, burdock (*Arctium lappa*), milk thistle (*Silybum marianum*), nettle (*Urtica dioica*), milky oat (*Avena sativa*), rose (*Rosa* spp.) hips

* At-risk botanicals: please research herbs before harvesting or purchasing and seek out potential substitutes or sustainably harvested or cultivated sources.

Summer is the season when energy is at its height. While we can ride this wave by embracing new projects, adding extra responsibilities to our plate, and connecting with others more frequently, we need to remember to keep ourselves nourished so we don't burn out. This season is the ideal time to eat a wide variety of whole foods to ensure adequate nutrition, incorporate culinary botanicals into meals to support digestion, and keep the body hydrated with plenty of water and cooling herbal teas. Sour flavors from fruits and herbs are plentiful this time of the year and are quite beneficial in keeping our hydration levels on track and supporting the tissues that line the digestive tract. These tart flavors often have an astringent action, helping to tighten and tone tissues, ensuring their proper function as a barrier so they allow certain nutrients to pass into the bloodstream while keeping other things out.

As we find ourselves more active, whether physically or mentally, during the summer, it's easy for our environment to take a toll on our bodies. This might mean we need to pay special care to our skin, muscles, and joints and keep ourselves hydrated, or it might look like taking periodic breaks to cool and calm an overstimulated mind and body.

Here , you will find several issues one might face during the summer season, along with recipes for herbal preparations that can be of assistance.

SUNBURN SPRITZER

Tend to overly hot summer skin that has been a little too kissed by the sun with a cooling botanical spritzer that not only cools skin upon contact but helps to ease inflammation and pain and stimulate cellular repair at the same time.

YIELD: 2 CUPS (480 ML)

Ingredients

1 cup (240 mL) water

2 tbsp (4 g) chamomile (*Matricaria chamomilla*) flower

1 tbsp (1 g) calendula (*Calendula officinalis*) flower

1 tbsp (2 g) comfrey (*Symphytum officinale*) leaf

1 tbsp (2 g) plantain (*Plantago* spp.) leaf

1 cup (240 mL) aloe (*Aloe vera*) juice

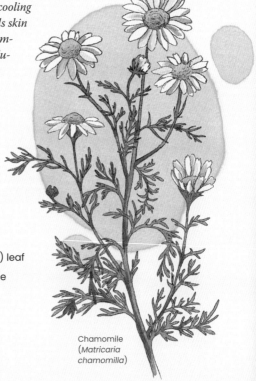

Chamomile (*Matricaria chamomilla*)

Aloe is an easy-to-grow houseplant and quite useful to have around for internal and external skin and mucous membrane needs. Just make sure you're growing an edible variety that is labeled *Aloe vera* or *Aloe barbadensis* (or a combination of these names). Edible aloe has thick gray-green leaves that form a rosette leaf pattern and produce yellow flowers when mature, where non-edible aloe has thinner white-flecked green leaves that form a stacked rosette or alternate leaf pattern and produce orange flowers when mature.

Directions

1 Bring 1 cup (240 mL) of water to a boil in a kettle or a small saucepan over medium-high heat. As soon as the water comes to a boil, remove it from the heat.

2 While the water is coming to a boil, combine herbs together in a quart-sized glass canning jar.

3 Pour 1 cup (240 mL) of boiled water over the ingredients, cap, and set the jar aside to infuse for 20 minutes or up to 4 hours (or overnight for a long-steep infusion).

4 When time is up, carefully strain the mixture through a fine-mesh sieve (lined with a few layers of cheesecloth to remove any plant material, if you wish). Press the herbs with the back of a spoon (or gather the edges of the cheesecloth to create a bundle and gently squeeze) to extract as much liquid as possible. Reserve the liquid in a clean glass storage container and compost the used plant material.

5 Add aloe juice to the herbal infusion and stir with a spoon to mix the two liquids together.

6 Transfer the liquid to a labeled glass storage bottle and cap with a spray top. Place additional liquid in an ice cube tray and freeze for later use.

Usage

Spritz over sun-kissed skin as often as needed to cool, moisturize, and soothe irritated skin.

Storage & Shelf-life

Store in the refrigerator for no more than 24 hours before making a fresh batch. Frozen ice cubes may be transferred to a glass storage container and stored for up to 6 months. When you are ready to use them, transfer the frozen ice cubes to a clean glass storage container and allow them to thaw in the refrigerator or at room temperature before transferring the liquid to a glass storage bottle and cap with a spray top.

BURN EASE PASTE

Blisters and burns are bound to happen. After initially cooling the burn site, this herbal paste can further support damaged tissue by protecting the site, calming inflammation and pain, and decreasing the chance of an infection forming.

YIELD: ½ CUP (120 ML)

Ingredients

3 tbsp (6 g) burdock (*Arctium lappa*) leaf

2 tbsp (4 g) plantain (*Plantago* spp.) leaf

1 tbsp (2 g) comfrey (*Symphytum officinale*) leaf

1 tbsp (2 g) lobelia (*Lobelia inflata*) aerial parts

1 tbsp (2 g) lavender (*Lavandula* spp.) flower bud

2 tbsp (30 mL) raw honey

2 tbsp (30 mL) aloe (*Aloe vera*) gel

60 drops of lavender (*Lavandula angustifolia*) essential oil (optional)

Burdock
(*Arctium lappa*)

You can create your own aloe gel by scraping the inner gel out of fresh aloe leaves and blending it in a blender. This should be stored in an air-tight dark-colored glass container in the refrigerator for no more than one week. You can also extend the shelf-life of fresh aloe by scraping the inner flesh out of the leaf, cutting it into chunks, and freezing the pieces on a baking sheet lined with natural waxed paper. Once frozen, these chunks can be stored together in a glass storage jar in the freezer for up to 12 months, allowing you to remove individual chunks of aloe as needed.

Directions

1 Measure each herb and combine together in a small coffee grinder to grind into a powder.

2 Sift the powder through a fine-mesh sieve, reserving the fine powder in a clean bowl and composting the larger plant material that remains in the sieve.

3 Add raw honey and aloe gel to the herbal powders, and mix well with a spoon until a paste forms.

4 If using, add 60 drops of lavender essential oil to the paste to create a 10% dilution, which is the suggested dilution for minor burns and acute injuries that do not need immediate medical attention.

5 Add additional liquids, if needed, to thin the paste, making it easier to apply to the skin. Transfer the paste to a labeled glass storage container. Cap and store for future use.

Usage

After cooling the burn site in lukewarm water, use a tongue depressor or popsicle stick to stir the paste to re-incorporate materials. Gently apply the paste to the burned skin covering the entire area. Cover with a piece of fresh burdock leaf (or another smooth leaf, such as plantain, comfrey, or violet) to create a non-stick barrier before applying a bandage to the site. Repeat this process every 12 hours until the burn heals.

Storage & Shelf-life

If using fresh aloe gel with no preservatives, store the burn paste in the refrigerator for 1–2 weeks before making a fresh batch. If using an aloe gel with preservatives, store the paste in the refrigerator for 6 months before making a fresh batch.

BRUISE–BE–GONE LINIMENT

Bruises hurt and are unsightly, so why not try to reduce your chances of a bruise forming after an injury or decrease the duration of a bruise if it does? With the help of botanicals that move stagnant or congealed blood, you can ease the pain, inflammation, swelling, and bruising associated with traumatic injuries, such as fractures, sprains, and contusions. For external use only! Do not use on broken skin!

YIELD: VARIES

Ingredients

2 parts arnica (*Arnica* spp.) flower tincture

1 part lavender (*Lavandula* spp.) flower bud tincture

1 part witch hazel (*Hamamelis virginiana*) bark tincture

Directions

1 Make individual tinctures following directions on pages 35–38.

2 When you are ready to create the liniment, choose the measurement you'd like to use for your part.

3 Measure out each tincture individually before combining them in a clean, labeled glass storage container. Cap and store for future use.

Usage

Apply a small amount of liniment to a cotton ball or clean cloth. Gently rub over the injured area 3–4 times a day.

Storage & Shelf-life

Store in a cool, dark location. Use within 3–5 years before making a fresh batch.

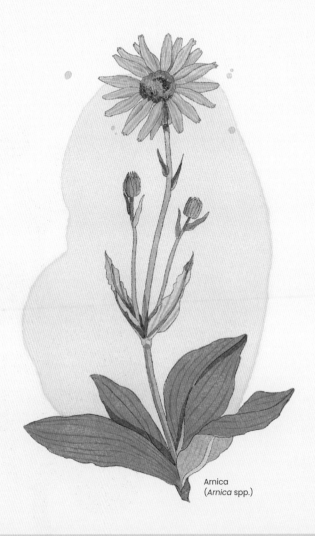

Arnica
(*Arnica* spp.)

Witch hazel is a deciduous tree or shrub that grows 5–15 feet tall. It blooms fragrant, yellow flowers after the leaves fade in late fall or early winter. Both the leaves and bark can be harvested and used for its astringent qualities. Leaves should be harvested in summer, while bark should be harvested in late autumn or early winter when the tannin content is the highest.

Herbal Electrolyte Tea

Stay hydrated in summer's heat (or when sickness arrives) with a tasty mineral-rich botanical infusion designed to replenish electrolytes lost through increased sweating, breathing heavily, vomiting and diarrhea, or other types of fluid loss.

YIELD: 2 CUPS (480 ML)

Ingredients

2 cups (480 mL) water

2 tbsp (3–4 g) Summer Days tea blend (below)

⅛ tsp (1 g) of Celtic sea salt

1–3 tsp (5–15 mL) raw honey (optional)

Summer Days Tea Blend:

3 parts hibiscus (*Hibiscus sabdariffa*) calyx

2 parts nettle (*Urtica dioica*) leaf

2 parts oat (*Avena sativa*) straw

1 part violet (*Viola* spp.) leaf

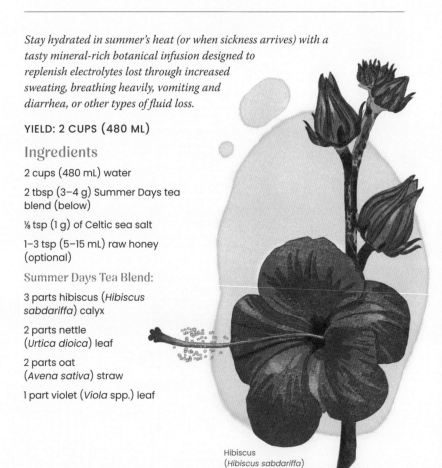

Hibiscus
(*Hibiscus sabdariffa*)

Celtic sea salt contains a wide variety of minerals and trace minerals and is a great way to support electrolyte balance in the body. You can also use cell salts or other electrolyte replacement options if you prefer.

Directions

1 Start by blending your Summer Days tea blend together. Measure out each herb individually and combine them in a large mixing bowl, stirring the herbs well to fully blend them together. Transfer this tea blend to a labeled glass storage container. Cap and store for future use.

2 When you are ready to make your electrolyte drink, bring 2 cups (480 mL) of water to a boil in a kettle or a small saucepan over medium-high heat. As soon as the water comes to a boil, remove it from the heat.

3 While the water is coming to a boil, combine 2 tbsp of Summer Days tea blend and ⅛ tsp of Celtic sea salt together in a pint-sized glass canning jar.

4 Pour 2 cups (480 mL) of boiled water over the ingredients, cap, and set aside to infuse for 20 minutes or up to 4 hours (or overnight for a long-steep infusion).

5 When time is up, carefully strain the mixture through a fine-mesh sieve lined with an unbleached coffee filter to remove any fine particles. Press the herbs with the back of a spoon (or gather the edges of the coffee filter to create a bundle and gently squeeze) to extract as much liquid as possible. Reserve the liquid in a clean, heat-proof mug or glass canning jar and compost the used plant material. Sweeten with raw honey, if desired.

Usage

Sip regularly throughout the day to maintain hydration and minerals. Enjoy up to 8 cups (1.9 L) a day, hot or cold.

Storage & Shelf-life

Store tea blend in a cool, dark location. Use within 12 months before making a fresh batch. Store prepared electrolyte tea in the refrigerator. Use within 24 hours before making a fresh batch.

Tip

• Feel free to make a cup of Summer Days tea (with or without the added electrolytes) to enjoy over ice during the summer months for a refreshing drink that will help keep you cool and nourished.

QUEASE–EASE SYRUP

Whether you're queasy from motion sickness during a summer road trip or from an unexpected illness, this herbal syrup will come to your aid to reduce feelings of nausea and upset stomach with the support of botanicals that help calm uncomfortable spasms in the digestive tract.

YIELD: 2 CUPS (480 ML)

Ingredients

¼ cup (56 g) fresh ginger (*Zingiber officinale*) rhizome, grated

2 cups (480 mL) water

1 cup (240 mL) raw honey

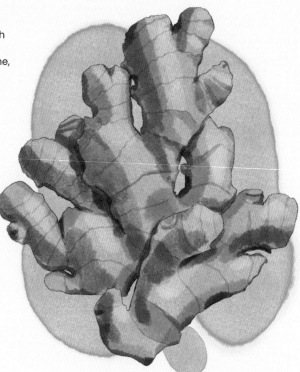

Ginger (*Zingiber officinale*)

Directions

1 Grate and measure ginger. Place it in a small saucepan with 2 cups (480 mL) of water and stir the mixture well to fully saturate the herbs with water.

2 Place the saucepan on the stove and bring the mixture to a boil over medium-high heat. When the water comes to a boil, immediately reduce the heat to a simmer. Allow the mixture to simmer until the water level has reduced by half—to 1 cup (240 mL)—to create a decoction.

3 Once the water level has reduced to 1 cup (240 mL), carefully strain the decoction through a fine-mesh sieve (lined with a few layers of cheesecloth to remove any plant material, if you wish). Press the herbs with the back of a spoon (or gather the edges of the cheesecloth to create a bundle and gently squeeze) to extract as much liquid as possible. Reserve the decocted liquid in a clean glass measuring cup, adding more water, if needed, to bring the total volume of liquid up to 1 cup (240 mL), and compost the used plant material.

4 Allow the liquid to cool slightly before adding 1 cup (240 mL) of raw honey. Stir well to combine and transfer to a labeled glass storage container. Cap and store for future use.

Usage

Take 1 tbsp (15 mL) of syrup up to 3 times a day. Take it straight off the spoon, mix it with seltzer water, or add it to a smoothie or yogurt bowl.

Storage & Shelf-life

Store syrup in the refrigerator. Use within 3–4 weeks before making a fresh batch.

Slow Down Styptic Powder

Slow bleeding from wounds through the astringent property of herbs, which helps to tighten and tone tissues, thus slowing bleeding until the blood can clot. When used externally, these herbs are called styptics, and they are a must-have for any herbal first-aid kit.

YIELD: VARIES

Ingredients

1 part yarrow (*Achillea millefolium*) leaf

1 part oak (*Quercus* spp.) bark

1 part plantain (*Plantago* spp.) leaf

Directions

1　Measure each herb and combine together in a small coffee grinder to grind into a powder.

2　Sift the powder through a fine-mesh sieve, reserving the fine powder in a labeled glass storage container and composting the larger plant material that remains in the sieve. Cap and store for future use.

Usage

Sprinkle powder in and on the bleeding wound. Place a clean cloth or gauze over the wound and apply firm pressure for 5–10 minutes, depending on the size of the wound, until the bleeding stops. Next, gently clean the wound with Wound Wash Tincture on page 96, doing your best to rinse powder and debris away, followed by gently drying and applying Wound-a-Way Herbal Oil on page 98 before bandaging. If bleeding begins again during cleansing, apply more pressure and use more styptic powder, if needed, and repeat the cleansing process.

Storage & Shelf-life

Store in the freezer. Use within 6 months before making a fresh batch.

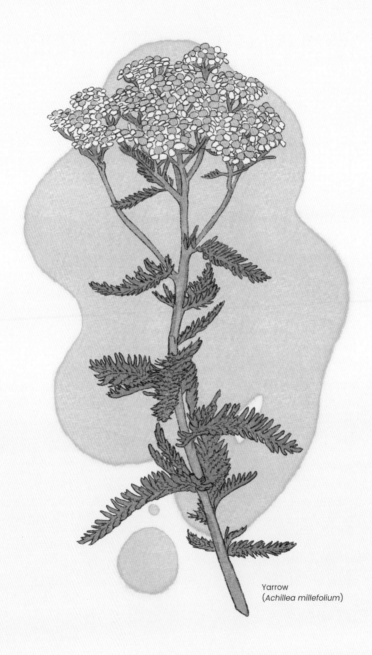

Yarrow
(*Achillea millefolium*)

WOUND WASH TINCTURE

Cuts, scraps, bites, stings, and lacerations are more likely during the warm days of summer when one is outdoors more often. Cleanse wounds, wash away debris, and minimize the chance of infection with the help of an herbal wound wash made from herbs known for their potent antimicrobial benefits. Not only is this easy to use, but it travels well, so you can bring it on all your summer outdoor adventures.

YIELD: VARIES

Ingredients

2 parts Oregon grape (*Berberis aquifolium*) root tincture**

1 part grindelia (*Grindelia* spp.) flower bud tincture

½ part clove (*Syzygium aromaticum*) bud tincture

** cultivated source

Directions

1 Make individual tinctures following directions on pages 35–38.

2 When you are ready to create the tincture blend, begin by choosing the measurement you'd like to use for your part.

3 Measure out each tincture individually before combining them in a clean, labeled glass storage container. Cap and store for future use.

Usage

Add 2–4 tsp (10–20 mL) of wound wash tincture to every 8 fl oz (240 mL) of warm (not hot) water. Mix well. Soak the wound in water for 15 minutes before drying, applying additional herbal preparations, and bandaging. Repeat up to 3 times a day.

Storage & Shelf-life

Store in a cool, dark location. Use within 3–5 years before making a fresh batch.

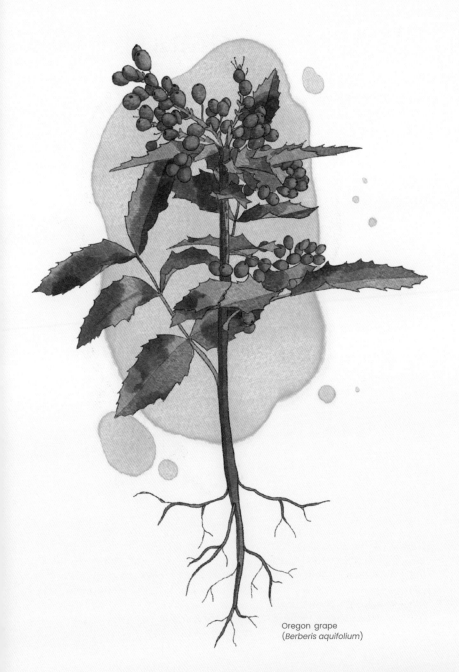

Oregon grape
(*Berberis aquifolium*)

WOUND-A-WAY HERBAL OIL

Stimulate tissue regeneration after wounds have been properly cleaned, helping them to repair themselves more quickly and efficiently, reducing the chance of infection and scarring by restoring your body's first defense against outside invaders—your skin!

YIELD: ½–1 CUP (120–240 ML)

Ingredients

½ cup (20 g) freshly wilted St. John's wort (*Hypericum perforatum*) aerial parts, packed

3 tbsp (6 g) yarrow (*Achillea millefolium*) aerial parts

4 tsp (4 g) chaparral (*Larrea tridentata*) aerial parts

½–1 cup (120-240 mL) olive oil

120-240 drops tea tree (*Melaleuca alternifolia*) essential oil (optional)

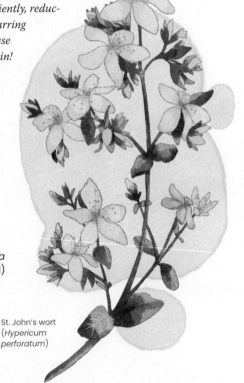

St. John's wort
(*Hypericum perforatum*)

The two constituents believed to be responsible for St. John's wort's ability to ease inflammation and nerve pain, deter microbial overgrowth, and stimulate tissue regeneration (amongst other beneficial actions) are hypericin and pseudohypericin. These phytochemicals are best extracted from fresh plant material rather than dried plant material. St. John's wort is a sturdy plant that has naturalized in many parts of the world and can grow in a variety of soils.

Directions

1 Begin by placing freshly harvested St. John's wort on a baking sheet lined with a cotton cloth or paper towels to wilt for 8–12 hours, which removes excess moisture from the plant material. Once the plant material has wilted, coarsely chop it to increase surface area exposure.

2 Measure all ingredients and follow the steps for the quick or slow herb-infused oil method on pages 32–34.

3 When your oil is finished, place a fine-mesh sieve (lined with a few layers of cheesecloth to remove plant material, if you wish) over a clean, dry glass container and carefully pour the mixture through it. Press the herbs with the back of a spoon (or gather the edges of the cheesecloth to create a bundle and gently squeeze) to extract as much liquid as possible. You can double strain the decanted liquid once more through a fine-mesh sieve lined with an unbleached coffee filter to further remove fine particles if you wish and compost the used plant material.

4 Use a glass measuring cup or graduated cylinder to measure the amount of herb-infused oil you have. If needed, add more olive oil to bring the total volume of oil back up to the amount you started with: ½–1 cup (120–240 mL).

5 If using, add 120 drops of tea tree essential oil for every ½ cup (120 mL) of herb-infused oil to create a 5% dilution, which is the suggested dilution for use on small surface areas of the skin during acute injuries.

6 Mix well with a spoon. Transfer the finished oil to a labeled glass storage container and allow it to cool completely. Once cool, cap and store for future use.

Usage

Apply a small amount of oil to cleaned wounds before bandaging. Repeat with each bandage change.

Storage & Shelf-life

Store in a cool, dark location. Use within 12 months before making a fresh batch.

Tip

• Substitute dried oregon grape (*Berberis aquifolium*) root** if you don't have access to fresh St. John's wort. ** cultivated source

Poison Ivy Ice Cubes

Poison ivy rashes range from irritating to unbearable depending on the level of exposure and sensitivity to the plant. Thankfully there are some herbal allies that can help protect the skin from developing a rash or lessening the extent of the rash upon exposure. They do this in a couple of ways, either by binding to the same molecular sites that the irritating oil in poison ivy binds or by binding to the oil itself, helping it be washed away more easily. Because fresh plant matter is most effective at the time of exposure, you can make poison ivy ice cubes to harness the beneficial properties of the fresh herb and use them any time of the year when you've been exposed to pesky poison ivy. It's best to choose a larger measurement for your parts in this recipe to ensure you end up with plenty of ice cubes.

YIELD: VARIES

Ingredients

2 parts fresh jewelweed (*Impatiens capensis, I. pallida*) aerial parts

2 parts fresh plantain (*Plantago* spp.) leaf

1 part fresh chickweed (*Stellaria media*) aboveground parts (optional)

1 part fresh violet (*Viola* spp.) leaf (optional)

Water or aloe (*Aloe vera*) gel/juice

Directions

1   Head outside to harvest fresh jewelweed and plantain, as well as chickweed and violet if you can find them growing in a cool, shady location. Rinse the plants under cool running water to wash away debris, and thoroughly shake them to remove excess water.

2   Roughly chop the plant material before measuring each herb using your chosen part. Then, place the measured plant material in a large bowl.

3   Begin by adding a small amount of fresh plant material and water in a high-speed blender and blending until a slurry forms. Gradually add more plant material (and additional water, if needed) until all plant material is well blended.

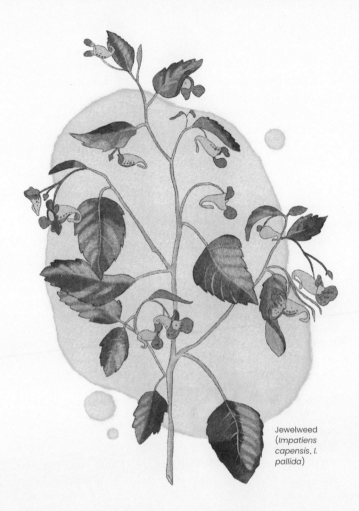

Jewelweed
(*Impatiens
capensis, I.
pallida*)

4 Once the mixture is blended, strain it through a fine-mesh sieve lined with
a few layers of cheesecloth to remove as much pulp as possible. Bundle the
cheesecloth and squeeze as much liquid as possible from the plant material
(which should be thick and slimy), reserving the liquid in a clean bowl, and
composting the used herbs.

5 Transfer the liquid to an ice cube tray and place it in the freezer overnight.
Once frozen, transfer the ice cubes to a labeled glass storage container. Cap
and store for future use.

Usage

After cleansing the skin with soap and cool water, rub an ice cube over the skin that was exposed to poison ivy to reduce the chance of developing a rash or minimize the severity of the rash. Leave the melted liquid on the skin for 15–20 minutes before rinsing with soap and cool water once more. Alternatively, you can melt the ice cube in a bowl before rubbing the liquid onto the skin.

Storage & Shelf-life

Store ice cubes in the freezer. Use within 6 months before making a fresh batch.

Jewelweed is one of the easiest herbs to identify. It grows in moist, shady areas in dense patches. It has knobby stems that are a translucent green in color with dark purple coloring where the plant branches. The stems are easy to break and contain a watery, mucilaginous liquid that is prized for reducing skin irritation. Its delicate leaves are thin and hairless, giving them a skin-like feel. Small bright orange or yellow flowers grow toward the top of the plant in summer and autumn, and its mature seed pods explode from the lightest touch, sending seeds flying in all directions, and giving the plant its common name "touch-me-not."

POISON IVY SPRAY

When a poison ivy rash develops, it can make a person miserable with itchy, weeping skin that is sometimes painful. Additionally, rashes are a break in the skin's protective barrier, and infections can sometimes develop. Using herbal allies with microbe-deterring and skin-protectant properties can help not only ease itching and dry the rash up more quickly but also help cleanse the skin and decrease the chances of infection.

YIELD: ½ CUP (120 ML)

Ingredients

4 tbsp (60 mL) grindelia (*Grindelia* spp.) flower bud tincture

2 tbsp (30 mL) plantain (*Plantago* spp.) leaf tincture

2 tbsp (30 mL) aloe (*Aloe vera*) juice

Directions

1 Measure and combine all ingredients in a labeled glass bottle and cap with a spray top.

2 Shake well to combine and store for future use.

Usage

Apply spray to rash 2–3 a day and allow to dry completely. Use on broken or sensitive skin may be irritating. Stop use if irritation occurs.

Storage & Shelf-life

Store in a cool, dark location. Use within 3–5 years before making a fresh batch.

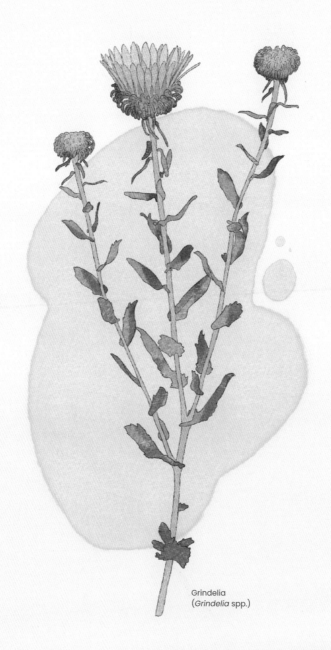

Grindelia
(*Grindelia* spp.)

ITCH EASE PASTE

Ease the itch of rashes with this simple oat and peppermint paste. Calming and cooling to the skin, this paste will not only soothe irritated skin but take your mind off the itch as well.

YIELD: ¾ CUP (180 ML)

Ingredients

½ cup (55 g) oat (*Avena sativa*) seed, rolled

¼ cup (8 g) peppermint (*Mentha x piperita*) leaf

Cold water

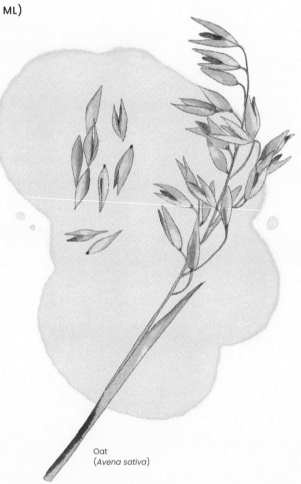

Oat
(*Avena sativa*)

Directions

1 Measure each herb and combine together in a small coffee grinder to grind into a powder.

2 Sift the powder through a fine-mesh sieve, reserving the fine powder in a labeled glass storage container and composting the larger plant material that remains in the sieve. Cap and store for future use.

3 When you are ready to make the paste, place 1 tbsp of powder into a glass bowl and add a small amount of cold water to it. Stir to combine, adding more water, if needed, until a paste forms that is the consistency of cake batter.

Usage

Spread the paste thinly over itchy rashes or bug bites and allow it to dry. Rinse the paste off with cool water and repeat as often as needed to ease itching and soothe skin.

Storage & Shelf-life

Store powder in a cool, dark location. Use within 12 months before making a fresh batch. Store excess paste in the refrigerator. Use within 24 hours before making a fresh batch.

Tip

• Add 1 cup of powder to a hot bath for all-over itch relief, mix well, and soak to relieve itching with heat.

An itching sensation is caused by a buildup of histamine in mast cells within the skin. Histamine is released when the skin is rubbed, but rubbing the skin leads to further irritation, pain, and chance of infection. Instead, histamine can also be released by changing the skin's temperature sensation by applying hot or cold things. Hot or cold compresses, ice cubes rubbed over the skin, or hot air from a blow dryer can all help to release histamine and ease itching without scratching.

SPLITTING HEADACHE TINCTURE

Heat sometimes has a way of bringing on a headache that feels like your head is going to split wide open. These types of headaches can be rooted in sickness accompanied by fever, too much time in the sun, not enough water, high blood pressure, or anything else that increases body temperature or blood flow within the body. Thankfully, there are cooling, relaxing herbs to come to our aid to help cool the body, disperse blood flow, and, most importantly, ease that splitting headache!

YIELD: VARIES

Ingredients

2 parts blue vervain (*Verbena hastata*) aerial parts tincture or glycerite

2 parts wood betony (*Betonica officinalis*) aerial parts tincture or glycerite

2 parts white willow (*Salix alba*) bark tincture or glycerite

1½ parts peppermint (*Mentha x piperita*) leaf tincture or glycerite

1½ parts skullcap (*Scutellaria lateriflora*) aerial parts tincture or glycerite

1 part licorice (*Glycyrrhiza glabra*) root tincture or glycerite

Directions

1 Make individual tinctures or glycerites following directions on pages 35–39.

2 Measure out each tincture or glycerite individually before combining them in a clean, labeled glass storage container. Cap and store for future use.

Usage

Take ½–1 tsp (2.5–5 mL) immediately, followed by ¼ tsp (1 mL) every 20–30 minutes for 2–3 hours, and then as needed for the remainder of the day.

Storage & Shelf-life

Store in a cool, dark location. Use within 3–5 years before making a fresh batch.

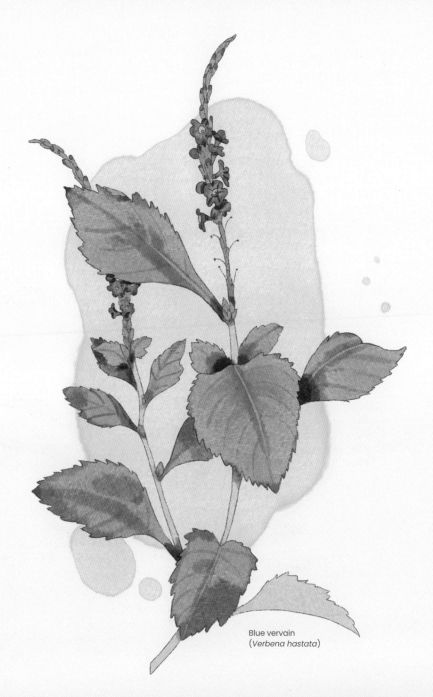

Blue vervain
(*Verbena hastata*)

Cooling Muscle Oil

Summer naturally encourages us to increase our activity level, which can sometimes lead to sore, achy, or tight muscles for a time. Thankfully, there are supportive allies that help to bring a cooling sensation to the tissues and soothe inflammation, ease achiness, and relax tension as well.

YIELD: ½–1 CUP (120–240 ML)

Ingredients

½ cup (28 g) eucalyptus (*Eucalyptus spp.*) leaf

¼ cup (4 g) arnica (*Arnica* spp.) aerial parts

½–1 cup (120–240 mL) olive oil

½–1 tsp (2–4 g) menthol crystals

24–48 drops of peppermint (*Mentha x piperita*) essential oil (optional)

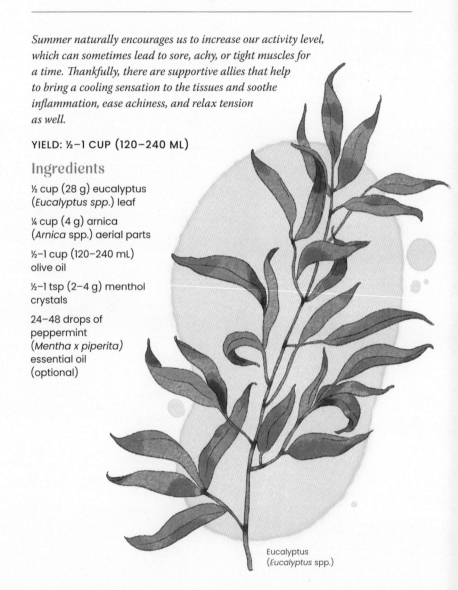

Eucalyptus
(*Eucalyptus* spp.)

Directions

1 Measure all ingredients and follow the steps for the quick or slow herb-infused oil method on pages 32–34.

2 When your oil is finished, place a fine-mesh sieve (lined with a few layers of cheesecloth to remove plant material, if you wish) over a clean, dry glass container and carefully pour the mixture through it. Press the herbs with the back of a spoon (or gather the edges of the cheesecloth to create a bundle and gently squeeze) to extract as much liquid as possible. You can double strain the decanted liquid once more through a fine-mesh sieve lined with an unbleached coffee filter to further remove fine particles if you wish and compost the used plant material.

3 Use a glass measuring cup or graduated cylinder to measure the amount of herb-infused oil you have. If needed, add more olive oil to bring the total volume of oil back up to the amount you started with: ½–1 cup (120–240 mL).

4 Transfer the strained herb-infused oil to a saucepan and add ½ to 1 tsp of menthol crystals, depending on how strong you want the menthol to be in the final oil. Heat over low heat, stirring frequently, until the crystals melt.

5 If using, add 24 drops of peppermint essential oil for every ½ cup (120 mL) of herb-infused oil to create a 1% dilution, which is the suggested dilution for stronger essential oils that are applied to larger surface areas of the body, especially when combined with menthol crystals.

6 Mix well with a spoon. Transfer the finished oil to a labeled glass storage container and allow it to cool completely. Once cool, cap and store for future use.

Usage

Apply a small amount of oil to sore or tight muscles, gently massage into the skin, and add more oil if needed. Repeat 3–4 times a day. For external use only!

Storage & Shelf-life

Store in a cool, dark location. Use within 12 months before making a fresh batch.

Tip

• Warming Winter Oil on page 188 or Spicy Salve on page 172 can feel great on sore muscles if you prefer a little heat.

Busted Joint Tincture

Sprains, strains, twists, and tweaks can happen to ankles and other joints during the summer months when activity levels are up, so having a supportive herbal tincture on hand can help to calm inflammation, increase blood flow, stimulate immune cells, increase lymphatic flow, and ease pain—all things that are great for those busted joints.

YIELD: VARIES

Ingredients

2 parts echinacea (*Echinacea angustifolia, E. purpurea*)
root tincture or glycerite**

2 parts willow (*Salix* spp.) bark tincture or glycerite

1 part ginger (*Zingiber officinale*) rhizome tincture or glycerite

½ part cayenne (*Capsicum annuum*) fruit tincture or glycerite

** cultivated source

Directions

1 Make individual tinctures or glycerites following directions on pages 35–39.

2 When you are ready to create the tincture or glycerite blend, begin by choosing the measurement you'd like to use for your part.

3 Measure out each tincture or glycerite individually before combining them in a clean, labeled glass storage container. Cap and store for future use.

Usage

Take ½–1 tsp (2.5–5 mL) 3 times a day until symptoms of joint injury have passed.

Storage & Shelf-life

Store in a cool, dark location. Use within 3–5 years before making a fresh batch.

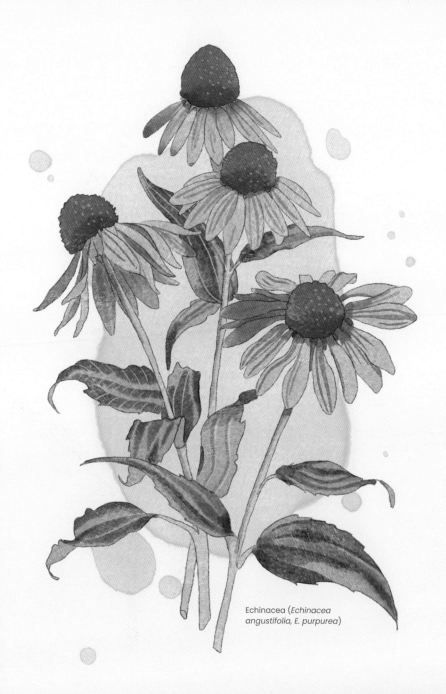

Echinacea (*Echinacea angustifolia, E. purpurea*)

Sprain Away Salve

Support tissue repair and ease inflammation when twisted ankles occur with an herb-infused salve packed with botanical allies known for their beneficial effects on soft tissues. These botanicals even help to disperse stagnant blood, which leads to bruising in injured tissue, helping bruises fade faster. For external use only!

YIELD: ½–1 CUP (120–240 ML)

Ingredients

½ cup (20 g) comfrey
(*Symphytum officinale*) leaf

½ cup (8 g) arnica
(*Arnica* spp.) aerial parts

½–1 cup (120–240 mL)
olive oil

¼–½ cup (28–56 g)
beeswax, grated or
pastille

72–144 drops of pine
(*Pinus* spp.) essential
oil (optional)

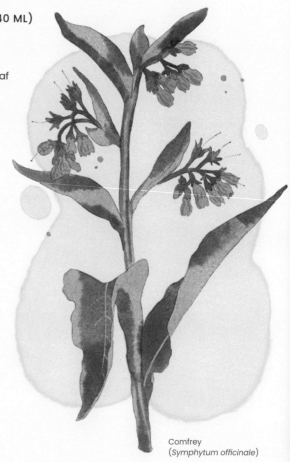

Comfrey
(*Symphytum officinale*)

Directions

1 Measure all ingredients and follow the steps for the quick or slow herb-infused oil method on pages 32–34.

2 When your oil is finished, place a fine-mesh sieve (lined with a few layers of cheesecloth to remove plant material, if you wish) over a clean, dry glass container and carefully pour the mixture through it. Press the herbs with the back of a spoon (or gather the edges of the cheesecloth to create a bundle and gently squeeze) to extract as much liquid as possible. You can double strain the decanted liquid once more through a fine-mesh sieve lined with an unbleached coffee filter to further remove fine particles if you wish and compost the used plant material.

3 When you are ready to make the salve, use a glass measuring cup or graduated cylinder to measure the amount of herb-infused oil you have. If needed, add more olive oil to bring the total volume of oil back up to the amount you started with: ½–1 cup (120–240 mL).

4 Next, measure out ¼ cup (28 g) of beeswax for every ½ cup (120 mL) of herb-infused oil you have. Place the beeswax into a clean saucepan, and heat it over medium-low heat until it has melted.

5 Turn the heat to low and pour the herb-infused oil into the saucepan alongside the melted beeswax. Carefully mix the two together until they're thoroughly combined.

6 Test the consistency of the salve by dipping a spoon in the mixture and letting it cool for a few minutes before touching it to get a feel for the final consistency. The goal is for the texture to be soft and easy to press. If the mixture is too hard, add a bit more oil. If the mixture is too soft, add another 1 tbsp (7 g) of beeswax. Be sure to go slow and make small adjustments, testing after each addition and repeating until you get the salve to the desired consistency.

7 Remove the saucepan from the heat and carefully transfer the mixture to a labeled tin or glass storage container.

8 If using, add 72 drops of pine essential oil for every ½ cup (120 mL) of herb-infused oil to create a 3% dilution, which is the suggested dilution for use on small surface areas of the body during acute injury. Stir the mixture with a toothpick and allow it to cool completely. Once cool, cap and store for future use.

Usage

Gently massage a small amount of salve into the skin as often as needed.

Storage & Shelf-life

Store in a cool, dark location. Use within 12 months before making a fresh batch.

Tip

- To test the consistency of your salve before transferring it to a storage container, dip a spoon in the liquid mixture and place it in the refrigerator to cool quickly. If the salve is too soft, add a bit more wax to the saucepan. If the salve is too hard, add a bit more of the reserved herb-infused oil. Repeat the test until you get the consistency you desire, and then transfer to your storage container.

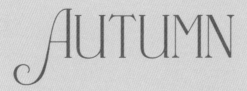

AUTUMN

Perhaps it's the trees adorned in shades of amber and crimson, the crisp breezes and gentle rustling of leaves underfoot, or the amber glow of the harvest moon and warm, cozy sweaters that make fall my favorite season of the year. After the long and busy days of summer, thoughts of stocking my home apothecary and preparing for the coming winter season are at the forefront of my mind. The plants are busy completing their life cycle—producing final fruits and developing seeds that will be left behind to bring forth the next generation, and I must carry on gathering and working with the botanical gifts nature continues to provide.

Throughout autumn, while the remains of late summer berries and seeds continue to be collected, the primary focus turns to harvesting sweet, nutrient-rich roots, which are available to gather as soon as the first frost kisses the earth.

Depending on your location and climate, some common herbs you might find during the autumn season include:

- Berries: sumac (*Rhus* spp.)
- Seeds: black walnut (*Juglans nigra*) hull, burdock (*Arctium lappa*), echinacea* (*Echinacea* spp.), milk thistle (*Silybum marianum*), rose (*Rosa* spp.) hip, yellow dock (*Rumex crispus*)
- Roots: angelica (*Angelica archangelica*), ashwagandha (*Withania somnifera*), astragalus (*Astragalus mongholicus*), black cohosh* (*Actaea racemosa*), blue cohosh* (*Caulophyllum thalictroides*), burdock (*Arctium lappa*), chicory (*Cichorium intybus*), codonopsis (*Codonopsis pilosula*), dandelion (*Taraxacum officinale*), echinacea* (*Echinacea* spp.), elecampane (*Inula helenium*), ginger (*Zingiber officinale*), goldenseal* (*Hydrastis canadensis*), gravel root (*Eutrochium purpureum*), horseradish (*Armoracia rusticana*), licorice (*Glycyrrhiza glabra*), marshmallow (*Althaea officinalis*), valerian (*Valeriana officinalis*), wild yam* (*Dioscorea villosa*), yellow dock (*Rumex crispus*)

* At-risk botanicals: please research herbs before harvesting or purchasing and seek out potential substitutes or sustainably harvested or cultivated sources.

While the shortening days and cooling weather of autumn signal us to spend time outdoors soaking up the last bit of light and warmth, it's almost as if the darkening days and falling leaves whisper subtle messages to us about accepting a slower pace of life, eventually finding ourselves bundling up, slowing down, and resting. This season brings about another transition in our diets as we shift once more toward warm, cooked foods that are often higher in starches and healthy fats. Sweet flavors from autumn roots, fruits, nuts, and spices are plentiful this time of year and provide deep nourishment for the cold seasons ahead. Not only are these foods quite beneficial to the gut, feeding beneficial bacteria that are so important to our overall health, but they also feed and nourish the nerves and endocrine systems, helping us to feel more grounded and centered during this seasonal transition.

In autumn, we find that our wellness focus shifts once again, only this time, our immune and endocrine systems are the body systems getting the majority of our attention. As the temperatures cool and the days darken, viral infections and external stressors tend to increase, leaving us feeling ill, depleted, or overwhelmed.

Here, you will find several issues one might face during autumn, along with a variety of herbal preparations that can be helpful throughout the season.

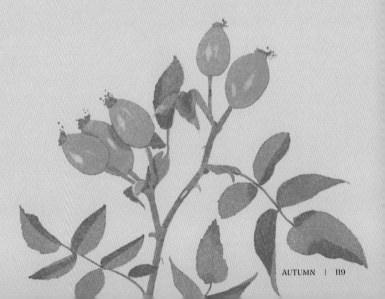

Immune Tonic Broth Blend

Give your immune system the support it needs to keep you healthy this fall with a blend of botanicals and fungi that can be added to your homemade broths and stocks to make them even healthier.

YIELD: VARIES

Ingredients

2 parts astragalus (*Astragalus mongholicus*) root

2 parts reishi (*Ganoderma* spp.) mushroom

2 parts burdock (*Arctium lappa*) root

1 part thyme (*Thymus vulgaris*) aerial parts

1 part parsley (*Petroselinum crispum*) leaf

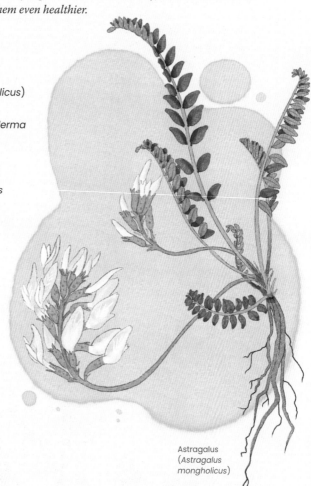

Astragalus
(*Astragalus mongholicus*)

Directions

1 Measure out each herb individually before combining them in a large mixing bowl, stirring the herbs well to incorporate them.

2 Transfer this mixture to a labeled glass storage container. Cap and store for future use.

Usage

Place 1 cup of broth blend in a layered cheesecloth (or a large cotton drawstring bag) and tie securely. Add 4 quarts (3.8 L) of water and other broth ingredients to a large pot. Bring the mixture to a boil, then reduce the heat and simmer for 3–4 hours (or longer for a more concentrated broth) before removing the bundle and straining the liquid.

Storage & Shelf-life

Store in a cool, dark location. Use within 12 months before making a fresh batch.

Tip

• Reuse the herbs in your broth blend by freezing the used bundle (cheese-cloth and all) until you're ready to make another batch of broth. When you're ready, simply add the frozen bundle to the pot and compost the herbs in the bundle after their second use.

Plant polysaccharides are beneficial to overall immune and gut health. These plant fibers act as prebiotics in the gut, feeding and increasing the number and variety of beneficial bacteria in the digestive tract. These bacteria and their metabolites then have positive effects on health and wellness, such as promoting anti-inflammatory activity, enhancing the intestinal barrier, and activating and regulating immune cells.

SCARBOROUGH CIDER

This milder cousin to Fire Cider still packs a punch where immune support is concerned. Made from aromatic, microbe-deterring culinary herbs that are easy to grow or source locally alongside raw apple cider vinegar and raw honey, this sweet and sour drink is a perfect addition to soups, sauces, broths and stocks, savory cocktails and mocktails, and more. Not to mention, a straight shot a day just might keep the doctor away!

YIELD: 2–3 QUARTS (2–3 L)

Ingredients

½ cup (14 g) thyme (*Thymus vulgaris*) aerial parts

¼ cup (20 g) rosemary (*Salvia rosmarinus*) leaf

¼ cup (10 g) sage (*Salvia officinalis*) leaf

¼ cup (3 g) parsley (*Petroselinum crispum*) leaf

1 large red onion (*Allium cepa*), chopped

3 heads garlic (*Allium sativum*), chopped

1 organic lemon (*Citrus* x *limon*) with peel, diced

2 tsp (5 g) black pepper (*Piper nigrum*) seeds, ground

Raw apple cider vinegar

Raw honey, to taste

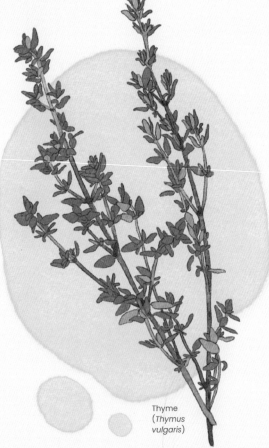

Thyme (*Thymus vulgaris*)

Directions

1 Measure out each ingredient individually and combine them in a half-gallon glass canning jar.

2 Pour raw apple cider vinegar over the plant material to cover it by 2–3 inches (5–8 centimeters). Place a piece of natural waxed paper between the jar and the lid to protect the contents from any chemicals that are on the lid.

3 Label the jar and place it in a warm location (like a seed-warming mat) for 2–3 weeks. Be sure to give the jar a shake every couple of days to keep the herbs and vinegar well-dispersed.

4 When time is up, open the jar and taste a bit of the liquid to see if the flavors of the plants are coming through. If you would like for it to be stronger, feel free to let it sit for a couple more weeks before straining, or transfer the contents of the jar to a high-speed blender and blend the batch, transferring it back to the glass canning jar to sit for another week or so.

5 When you are happy with the flavor, carefully pour the mixture through a fine-mesh sieve (lined with a few layers of cheesecloth to remove any plant material, if you wish). Press the herbs with the back of a spoon (or gather the edges of the cheesecloth to create a bundle and squeeze) to extract as much liquid as possible, and transfer the liquid to a bowl. If you previously blended the batch, it's a good idea to cover the strained liquid and let it sit on the counter overnight so any solid material settles to the bottom of the jar. In the morning, you can carefully pour off the clear liquid.

6 Once the liquid is filtered, add enough raw honey to the liquid to sweeten it to your liking. This may be ⅓–½ of the amount of liquid you have. Start with a small amount and taste the liquid after each addition, working your way up until your cider reaches a pleasing flavor.

7 Transfer the finished cider to a clean, labeled glass storage container. Cap and store for future use.

Usage

Take 1 tbsp (15 mL) daily as an immune or digestive aid. Increase to 3 tbsp (45 mL) daily during active infection or digestive upset.

Storage & Shelf-life

Store in a cool, dark location. Use within 6 months before making a fresh batch.

Tip

• Have fresh culinary herbs on hand? Simply double the measurements above when using fresh herbs. Store the finished product in the refrigerator and use it within 6 months before making a fresh batch.

Culinary herbs are easy to grow in containers! These aromatic plants flourish in pots, providing a fresh and convenient supply of flavorful additions to your culinary creations all year long. Whether you have a spacious backyard, a cozy balcony, or an indoor windowsill, growing culinary herbs in containers is a breeze due to minimal space requirements and simple care needs.

KID-FRIENDLY FIRE CIDER

Fire Cider is a cold and flu staple in many home apothecaries, but due to its spicy nature, it's rarely a favorite of the little ones. Thankfully, this classic immune-stimulating preparation is quite adaptable. Instead of hot and spicy botanicals, this version includes a bit of sweetness and spice and tastes oh, so nice! Packed with aromatic, microbe-deterring herbs, you'll certainly have less of a struggle getting your kids to take this version.

YIELD: 2–3 QUARTS (2–3 L)

Ingredients

1 cup (32 g) bee balm (*Monarda fistulosa*) aerial parts

½ cup (7 g) calendula (*Calendula officinalis*) flower

½ cup (112 g) fresh ginger (*Zingiber officinale*) rhizome, grated

5 sticks (25 g) cinnamon (*Cinnamomum verum*) bark, crushed

2 tbsp (12 g) clove (*Syzygium aromaticum*) bud

Raw apple cider vinegar

Raw honey, to taste

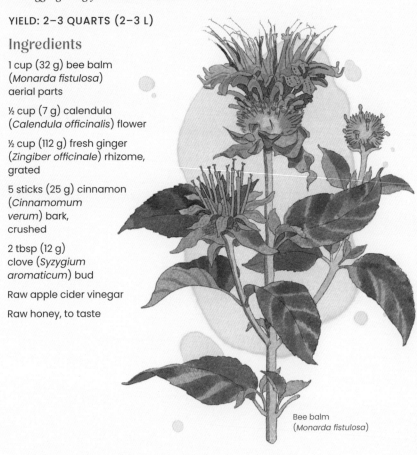

Bee balm
(*Monarda fistulosa*)

Directions

1 Measure out each ingredient individually and combine them in a half-gallon glass canning jar.

2 Pour raw apple cider vinegar over the plant material to cover it by 2–3 inches (5–8 centimeters). Place a piece of natural waxed paper between the jar and the lid to protect the contents from any chemicals that are on the lid.

3 Label the jar and place it in a warm location (like a seed-warming mat) for 2–3 weeks. Be sure to give the jar a shake every couple of days to keep the herbs and vinegar well-dispersed.

4 When time is up, open the jar and taste a bit of the liquid to see if the flavors of the plants are coming through. If you would like for it to be stronger, feel free to let it sit for a couple more weeks before straining, or transfer the contents of the jar to a high-speed blender and blend the batch, transferring it back to the glass canning jar to sit for another week or so.

5 When you are happy with the flavor, carefully pour the mixture through a fine-mesh sieve (lined with a few layers of cheesecloth to remove any plant material, if you wish). Press the herbs with the back of a spoon to extract as much liquid as possible, and transfer the liquid to a bowl. If you previously blended the batch, it's a good idea to cover the strained liquid and let it sit on the counter overnight so any solid material settles to the bottom of the jar. In the morning, you can carefully pour off the clear liquid.

6 Once the liquid is filtered, add enough raw honey to the liquid to sweeten it to your liking. This may be ⅓–½ of the amount of liquid you have. Start with a small amount and taste the liquid after each addition, working your way up until your cider reaches a pleasing flavor.

7 Transfer the finished cider to a clean, labeled glass storage container. Cap and store for future use.

Usage

Take 1–2 tsp (5–10 mL) daily as an immune or digestive aid. Increase to 1 tbsp (15 mL) daily during active infection or digestive upset.

Storage & Shelf-life

Store in a cool, dark location. Use within 6 months before making a fresh batch.

Tip

- If your child is sensitive to spicy flavors, feel free to reduce the amount of ginger, cinnamon, and clove to better suit their taste preferences. You can always add more, if needed, when you taste test in step 4.

Bee balm (also known as wild bergamot) is high in volatile oils and is well-known for its immune-supportive properties. This plant is native to North America and can be found growing wild in many parts of the country, as well as some parts of Europe. It's also quite easy to grow as long as it has well-drained soil and full sun to partial shade. Just remember, it's part of the mint family of plants, so it will spread easily. There are over 20 species of *Monarda* to choose from, and all species are used interchangeably. It comes in a variety of colors, blooming in late summer, making it a great fit for any garden.

BASIC, BETTER, BEST ELDERBERRY SYRUP

Antiques Road Show has nothing on this elderberry syrup contest, as each of the three is a valuable staple in the autumn apothecary. Depending on what ingredients you have on hand or how much immune support you want to add, these three elderberry syrup recipes will come to your aid when you've been exposed to a viral invader or come down with an active infection.

YIELD: 4 CUPS (960 ML)

Ingredients

Basic:

½ cup (55 g) elder (*Sambucus nigra, S. canadensis*) berry

4 cups (960 mL) water

2 cups (480 mL) raw honey

Better:

½ cup (55 g) elder (*Sambucus nigra, S. canadensis*) berry

2 tsp (10 g) fresh ginger (*Zingiber officinale*) rhizome, grated

1 stick (5 g) cinnamon (*Cinnamomum verum*) bark, crushed

1 tsp (2 g) clove (*Syzygium aromaticum*) bud

3 (1 g) cardamom (*Elettaria cardamomum*) pods, crushed

4 cups (960 mL) water

2 cups (480 mL) raw honey

Best:

½ cup (55 g) elder (*Sambucus nigra, S. canadensis*) berry

2 tsp (10 g) fresh ginger (*Zingiber officinale*) rhizome, grated

1 stick (5 g) cinnamon (*Cinnamomum verum*) bark, crushed

1 tsp (2 g) clove (*Syzygium aromaticum*) bud

3 (1 g) cardamom (*Elettaria cardamomum*) pods, crushed

1 tbsp (1 g) calendula (*Calendula officinalis*) flower

2 tsp (5 g) licorice (*Glycyrrhiza glabra*) root

4 cups (960 mL) water

2 cups (480 mL) raw honey

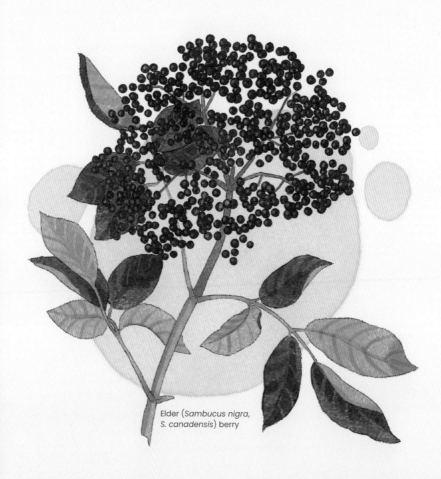

Elder (*Sambucus nigra,
S. canadensis*) berry

Elderberry has been a prized herb since ancient times and has been reported in modern scientific studies to prevent or reduce the severity of viral infections. Elder can be found growing in lush forests, in fields and meadows, and along creeks and streams. It's also a great herb to cultivate. Just make sure you have plenty of growing room. They can range from 10–30 feet tall and live for up to 60 years!

Directions

1 Measure herbs and combine them together in a small saucepan. Pour 4 cups (960 mL) of water over the plant material, stirring the mixture well to fully saturate the herbs with water, and place a lid on the saucepan. Allow this mixture to sit for 12–24 hours, giving the harder plant parts time to soften, if desired.

2 When you are ready to make the syrup, place the saucepan on the stove, remove the lid, and bring the mixture to a boil over medium-high heat. When the water comes to a boil, immediately reduce the heat to bring the mixture to a simmer and hold it there until the water level has reduced by half—to 2 cups (480 mL)—to create a decoction.

3 Once the water level has reduced to 2 cups (480 mL), carefully strain the decoction through a fine-mesh sieve (lined with a few layers of cheesecloth to remove any plant material, if you wish). Press the herbs with the back of a spoon (or gather the edges of the cheesecloth to create a bundle and squeeze) to extract as much liquid as possible. Reserve the decocted liquid in a clean glass measuring cup, adding more water, if needed, to bring the total volume of liquid up to 2 cups (480 mL), and compost the used plant material.

4 Allow the liquid to cool slightly before adding 2 cups (480 mL) of raw honey. Stir well to combine and transfer to a labeled glass storage container. Cap and store for future use.

Usage

Take 2–4 tbsp (30–60 mL) daily for 7 days after viral exposure to prevent infection. Increase to 2–4 tbsp (30–60 mL) every 2–4 hours at first sign of active infection until symptoms reside.

Storage & Shelf-life

Store in the refrigerator. Use within 3–4 weeks before making a fresh batch.

Tip

* Increase the shelf-life of your syrups to 1 year (unrefrigerated) when you add equal parts herbal decoction and food-grade vegetable glycerin or you add equal parts herbal decoction, honey, and tincture/alcohol.

HIGH C INFUSION

Vitamin C is the immune system's best friend. Not only does it support the production and function of immune cells, but it strengthens physical barriers against pathogens, supports tissue repair, and regulates the inflammatory response in the body—all important things when the body is dealing with an infection. Sipping this tart but tasty vitamin C–rich infusion over ice on warm autumn days is quite refreshing and a great way to provide your body with a regular supply of this valuable vitamin.

YIELD: 4 CUPS (960 ML)

Ingredients

4 cups (960 mL) water

¼ cup (13 g) High C infusion blend (below)

Raw honey, to taste (optional)

High C Infusion Blend:

3 parts hibiscus (*Hibiscus sabdariffa*) calyx

3 parts cinnamon (*Cinnamomum verum*) bark

2 parts violet (*Viola* spp.) leaf

2 parts tulsi (*Ocimum tenuiflorum*) aerial parts

1 part elder (*Sambucus nigra, S. canadensis*) berry

½ part rose (*Rosa* spp.) hip

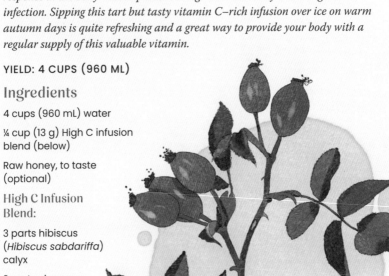
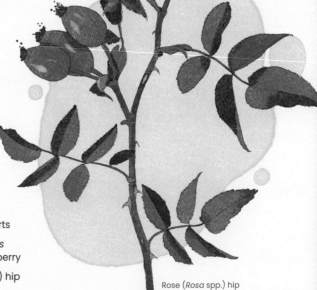

Rose (*Rosa* spp.) hip

Directions

1 Start by blending your High C infusion tea blend together. Measure out each herb individually and combine them in a large mixing bowl, stirring the herbs well to fully blend them together. Transfer this tea blend to a labeled glass storage container. Cap and store for future use.

2 When you are ready to make your tea, bring 4 cups (960 mL) of water to a boil using a kettle or a small saucepan over medium-high heat. As soon as the water comes to a boil, remove it from the heat and allow it to cool for 5–10 minutes to best preserve the vitamin C in the plant material.

3 While the water is coming to a boil, place ¼ cup of High C infusion blend in a quart-sized glass canning jar.

4 Pour 4 cups (960 mL) of boiled water over the plant material, cap, and set aside to infuse for 20 minutes or up to 4 hours (or overnight for a long-steep infusion).

5 When time is up, carefully strain the mixture through a fine-mesh sieve lined with an unbleached coffee filter to remove any fine particles. Press the herbs with the back of a spoon (or gather the edges of the coffee filter to create a bundle and gently squeeze) to extract as much liquid as possible. Reserve the liquid in a clean, heat-proof mug or glass canning jar and compost the used plant material. Sweeten with raw honey, if desired.

Usage

Drink up to 4 cups (960 mL) a day, hot or cold.

Storage & Shelf-life

Store infusion blend in a cool, dark location. Use within 12 months before making a fresh batch. Store the prepared infusion in the refrigerator until you're ready to drink it. Use within 24 hours before making a fresh batch.

ᴀᴛ Fɪʀsᴛ Sɪɢɴ Sʜᴏᴛs

No matter how much effort you put into preventing sickness, it will still happen sometimes. Thankfully, there are botanical allies that pack a powerful punch and can come to your aid when sickness rears its ugly head. These tiny but mighty herbal shots are meant to be taken at the first sign of sickness to stimulate the immune system and, hopefully, decrease the severity and duration of the illness.

YIELD: ½ CUP (120 ML)

Ingredients

¼ cup (60 mL) raw apple cider vinegar

¼ cup (60 mL) honey

¼ cup (56 g) fresh ginger (*Zingiber officinale*) rhizome, grated

1 stick (5 g) cinnamon (*Cinnamomum verum*) bark, crushed

1 small orange (or ½ large)

¼ tsp (2 g) sea salt

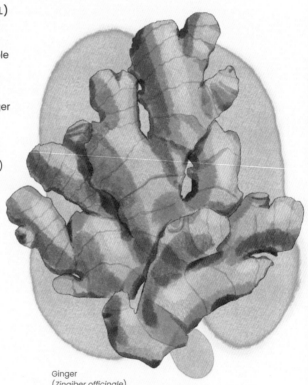

Ginger
(*Zingiber officinale*)

Directions

1 Combine all ingredients in a high-speed blender and blend for 10–15 minutes, keeping an eye on the blender base to make sure it doesn't get too hot.

2 Strain the mixture through a fine-mesh sieve (lined with a few layers of cheesecloth to remove plant material, if you wish), reserving the liquid in a clean glass jar. Press the herbs with the back of a spoon (or gather the edges of the cheesecloth to create a bundle and gently squeeze) to extract as much liquid as possible and compost the used plant material.

3 Taste the liquid and adjust the flavor to suit your preference by adding additional honey, if desired, until it suits your taste.

4 Transfer the liquid to a labeled glass container. Cap and store for future use.

Usage

Pour 1 fl oz (30 mL) into a cup and dilute with a bit of water or coconut water, if desired. Drink every 2 hours at the first sign of a viral infection.

Storage & Shelf-life

Store the mixture in the refrigerator, using it within 2–3 weeks before making a fresh batch.

Tip

• Ginger is a potent and effective herbal ally during viral infections, particularly when used right away when the first symptoms of illness begin to appear. I like to use ginger shots during the first 24 hours of a viral illness and then switch over to elderberry syrup for the remainder of the illness.

OH! MY ACHING HEAD TINCTURE

Colds, congestion, and sinus pressure from seasonal allergies or viral illnesses can contribute to a dull, aching headache that feels like it's throbbing inside your whole head! Thankfully there are warming, dispersive herbs that help move stagnant fluids and relax tension in the body, so you can ease your aching head as naturally as possible.

YIELD: VARIES

Ingredients

3 parts valerian (*Valeriana officinalis*) root tincture or glycerite

3 parts yarrow (*Achillea millefolium*) aerial parts tincture or glycerite

2 parts California poppy (*Eschscholzia californica*) aboveground parts tincture or glycerite

1½ parts lavender (*Lavandula* spp) flower bud tincture or glycerite

1 part sage (*Salvia officinalis*) leaf tincture or glycerite

½ part kava (*Piper methysticum*) root* tincture or glycerite

* sustainably sourced

Directions

1 Make individual tinctures or glycerites following directions on pages 35–39.

2 When you are ready to create the tincture or glycerite blend, begin by choosing the measurement you'd like to use for your part.

3 Measure out each tincture or glycerite individually before combining them in a clean, labeled glass storage container. Cap and store for future use.

Usage

Take ½–1 tsp (2.5–5 mL) immediately, followed by ¼ tsp (1 mL) every 20–30 minutes for 2–3 hours, and then as needed for the remainder of the day.

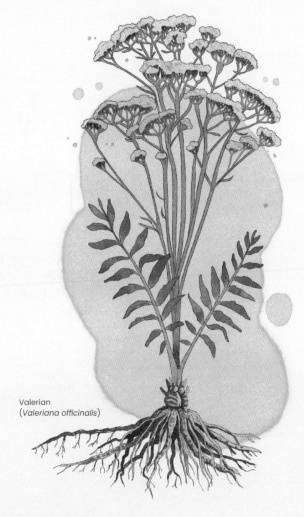

Valerian
(*Valeriana officinalis*)

Storage & Shelf-life

Store in a cool, dark location. Use within 3–5 years before making a fresh batch.

Sore Throat Pastilles

Ease the pain of sore, scratchy throats or spastic irritating coughs with these soothing herbal pastilles. Sweet and spicy (or cooling—you decide), these tiny herb pastilles are a tasty treat that feels so good to hot, dry tissues of the throat when you suck on them and let their demulcent, skin-soothing, inflammation-easing properties get to work.

YIELD: VARIES

Ingredients

2 parts marshmallow
(*Althaea officinalis*) root powder

1 part sage (*Salvia officinalis*)
leaf powder

1 part plantain (*Plantago* spp.)
leaf powder

Raw honey

Cinnamon
(*Cinnamomum verum*)
bark or peppermint
(*Mentha* x *piperita*) leaf
powder (for coating)

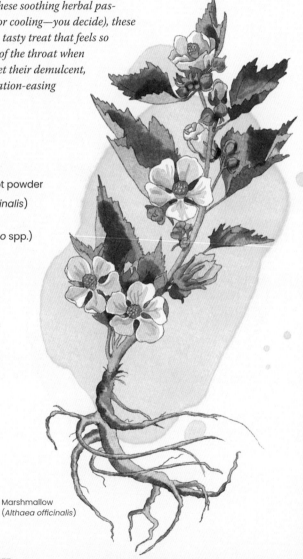

Marshmallow
(*Althaea officinalis*)

Directions

1 To begin, place a small amount of each individual herb in a small coffee grinder to grind into a powder. Sift the powder through a fine-mesh sieve, reserving the fine powder in a clean bowl (one bowl for each herbal powder) and composting the larger plant material that remains in the sieve.

2 When you are ready to make the pastilles, measure each herbal powder, combining them together in a large mixing bowl.

3 Add a small amount of honey to the powder and mix until a stiff dough forms. Adjust for consistency by adding more herbal powder to create a stiffer dough or more honey for a softer dough.

4 Once the dough is at the correct consistency to roll out little balls (pastilles), pinch off small pieces of dough and roll them into dime-sized balls. Transfer the dough balls into herbal powder to coat them. Cinnamon is tasty and warming, and peppermint is refreshing and cooling, but any flavorful herbal powder will work. Dust the dough balls in the coating powder and transfer them to a labeled glass storage container. Add some additional coating powder to the container to keep the pastilles from sticking to one another. Cap and store for future use.

Usage

Take 1 pastille anytime you feel your throat is dry or sore, letting it slowly dissolve in your mouth. Repeat as often as needed.

Storage & Shelf-life

Store in a cool, dark location. Use within 6 months before making a fresh batch.

Tip

• To make your own powders, place dried plant material, one herb at a time, in a coffee grinder. Set the grinder to a fine setting and grind for 30–60 seconds. Sift the ground plant material through a fine-mesh sieve reserving the fine powder in a bowl and composting the coarse plant material that remains in the sieve.

GOOT Ointment

Sore throat, cough, and chest congestion are common during the autumn months, particularly when cold and flu season arrives. These issues are generally mild and go away on their own, but for some, they can worsen quickly if not cared for properly. GOOT, which stands for garlic olive oil treatment, is a great way to support the body during these conditions. Not only does it feel good when massaged into the neck, chest, back, and bottoms of the feet, but it packs a bacteria-deterring punch that can help decrease the chance of any of these conditions from turning into a full-blown infection.

YIELD: ½ CUP (120 ML)

Ingredients

½ cup (120 mL) olive oil

5–6 (30 g) fresh garlic (*Allium sativum*) cloves, minced

3 tbsp (21 g) beeswax, grated or pastille

72 drops of tea tree (*Melaleuca alternifolia*) essential oil (optional)

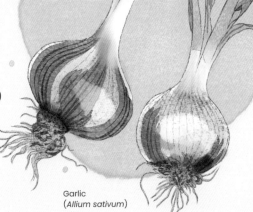

Garlic
(*Allium sativum*)

Directions

1 Measure all ingredients and follow the steps for the quick herb-infused oil method on pages 33–34.

2 When your oil is finished, place a fine-mesh sieve (lined with a few layers of cheesecloth to remove plant material, if you wish) over a clean, dry glass container and carefully pour the mixture through it. Press the herbs with the back of a spoon (or gather the edges of the cheesecloth to create a bundle and gently squeeze) to extract as much liquid as possible. You can double strain the decanted liquid once more through a fine-mesh sieve lined with an unbleached coffee filter to further remove fine particles if you wish and compost the used plant material.

3 When you are ready to make the ointment, use a glass measuring cup or graduated cylinder to measure the amount of herb-infused oil you have. If needed, add more olive oil to bring the total volume of oil back up to the amount you started with: ½ cup (120 mL).

4 Measure out 3 tbsp (21 g) of beeswax, add it into a clean saucepan, and heat it over medium-low heat until it has melted.

5 Turn the heat to low and pour the herb-infused oil into the saucepan alongside the melted beeswax. Carefully mix the two together until they're thoroughly combined.

6 Test the consistency of the ointment by dipping a spoon in the mixture and letting it cool for a few minutes before touching it to get a feel for the final consistency. The goal is for the texture to be soft and easy to press. If the mixture is too hard, add a bit more oil. If the mixture is too soft, add another 1 tbsp (7 g) of beeswax. Be sure to go slow and make small adjustments, testing after each addition and repeating until you get the ointment to the desired consistency.

7 Remove the saucepan from the heat and carefully transfer the mixture to a labeled tin or glass storage container.

8 If using, add 72 drops of tea tree essential oil to create a 3% dilution, which is the suggested dilution for use on small surface areas of the body during acute illness. Stir the mixture with a toothpick and allow it to cool completely. Once cool, cap and store for future use.

Usage

With a clean finger, scoop a small amount of ointment out of the storage container and massage it gently into the neck, chest, back, and bottoms of the feet as often as needed.

Storage & Shelf-life

Store in a cool, dark location. Use within 12 months before making a fresh batch.

Tip

- To adjust the consistency of the ointment, dip a spoon in the oil and wax mixture while in the saucepan and let it cool for a few minutes before touching it to get a feel for the final consistency. If the mixture is too firm, add a bit more herb-infused oil. If the mixture is too soft, add a bit more melted wax. Be sure to go slow and make small adjustments, testing after each addition, and repeating until you get the ointment to the consistency you prefer.

CALMING COUGH SYRUP

Constant, spastic-like, ticklish, or dry coughs can often be the most annoying types of cough because they seem to be never-ending and useless. Thankfully, there are some botanical allies that can help quell a cough, soothe and moisturize dry tissues, and calm irritation so you can spend less time coughing and more time doing what you'd like.

YIELD: 1–1½ CUP (240–360 ML)

Ingredients

3 tbsp (6 g) mullein (*Verbascum thapsus*) leaf

2 tbsp (3 g) violet (*Viola* spp.) leaf

2 tsp (6 g) licorice (*Glycyrrhiza glabra*) root

1 cup (240 mL) water

½ cup (120 mL) raw honey

½ cup (120 mL) wild cherry bark tincture (optional)

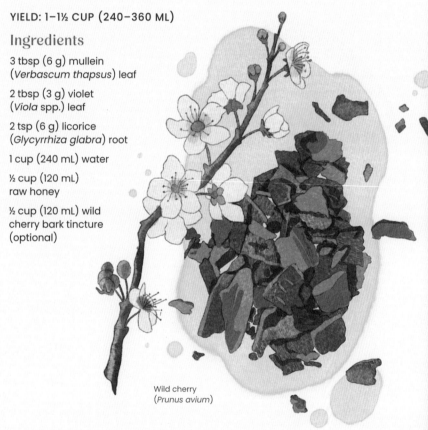

Wild cherry
(*Prunus avium*)

Directions

1 Measure herbs and combine them together in a small saucepan. Pour 1 cup (240 mL) of water over the plant material, stirring the mixture well to fully saturate the herbs with water, and place a lid on the saucepan. Allow this mixture to sit for 12–24 hours, giving the harder plant parts time to soften, if desired.

2 When you are ready to make the syrup, place the saucepan on the stove, remove the lid, and bring the mixture to a boil over medium-high heat. When the water comes to a boil, immediately reduce the heat to bring the mixture to a simmer and hold it there until the water level has reduced by half—to ½ cup (120 mL)—to create a decoction.

3 Once the water level has reduced to ½ cup (120 mL), carefully strain the decoction through a fine-mesh sieve (lined with a few layers of cheesecloth to remove any plant material, if you wish). Press the herbs with the back of a spoon (or gather the edges of the cheesecloth to create a bundle and squeeze) to extract as much liquid as possible. Reserve the decocted liquid in a clean glass measuring cup, adding more water, if needed, to bring the total volume of liquid up to ½ cup (120 mL), and compost the used plant material.

4 Allow the liquid to cool slightly before adding ½ cup (120 mL) of raw honey and ½ cup (120 mL) of tincture, if using. Stir well to combine and transfer to a labeled glass storage container. Cap and store for future use.

Usage

Take 1–2 tsp (5–10 mL) every 2–4 hours.

Storage & Shelf-life

Store in a cool, dark location. Use syrups made without a tincture within 3–4 weeks and use syrups made with a tincture within 12 months before making a fresh batch.

Wild cherry bark should be harvested from small branches taken directly from the tree—never from fallen branches. Once the branch is detached from the tree, the bark begins to ferment and becomes toxic due to the conversion of cyanogenic glycosides within the bark into hydrocyanic acid. Freshly harvested bark should be dried immediately and completely before storing for future use.

Up and Out Cough Syrup

Some coughs are quite loud and loose due to excess mucous in the lungs. These types of coughs seem to build up over time, eventually causing you to have to cough to get all of that loose mucous up and out. Why not encourage your body to dry up all that excess mucous through the help of aromatic, microbe-deterring herbs so you can not only support your immune and respiratory systems but also get back to normal a bit faster?

YIELD: 1–1½ CUPS (240–360 ML)

Ingredients

¼ cup (10 g) sage (*Salvia officinalis*) leaf

2 tbsp (6 g) hyssop (*Hyssopus officinalis*) leaf

1 cup (240 mL) water

½ cup (120 mL) raw honey

½ cup (120 mL) anise (*Pimpinella anisum*) seed tincture (optional)

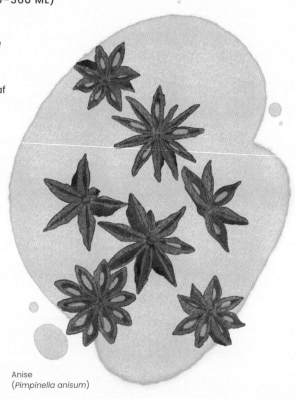

Anise
(*Pimpinella anisum*)

Directions

1 Measure herbs and combine them together in a small saucepan. Pour 1 cup (240 mL) of water over the plant material, stirring the mixture well to fully saturate the herbs with water, and place a lid on the saucepan. Allow this mixture to sit for 12–24 hours, giving the harder plant parts time to soften, if desired.

2 When you are ready to make the syrup, place the saucepan on the stove, remove the lid, and bring the mixture to a boil over medium-high heat. When the water comes to a boil, immediately reduce the heat to bring the mixture to a simmer and hold it there until the water level has reduced by half—to ½ cup (120 mL)—to create a decoction.

3 Once the water level has reduced to ½ cup (120 mL), carefully strain the decoction through a fine-mesh sieve (lined with a few layers of cheesecloth to remove any plant material, if you wish). Press the herbs with the back of a spoon (or gather the edges of the cheesecloth to create a bundle and squeeze) to extract as much liquid as possible. Reserve the decocted liquid in a clean glass measuring cup, adding more water, if needed, to bring the total volume of liquid up to ½ cup (120 mL), and compost the used plant material.

4 Allow the liquid to cool slightly before adding ½ cup (120 mL) of raw honey and ½ cup (120 mL) of tincture, if using. Stir well to combine and transfer to a labeled glass storage container. Cap and store for future use.

Usage

Take 1–2 tsp (5–10 mL) every 2–4 hours.

Storage & Shelf-life

Store in a cool, dark location. Use syrups made without a tincture within 3–4 weeks and use syrups made with a tincture within 12 months before making a fresh batch.

LOOSEN UP COUGH SYRUP

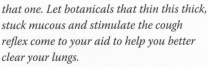

Perhaps the most frustrating kind of cough is one that's tight, tense, and heavy. You know, the one that feels like there's something stuck deep in your chest, but you just can't seem to get it up and out? Yeah, that one. Let botanicals that thin this thick, stuck mucous and stimulate the cough reflex come to your aid to help you better clear your lungs.

YIELD: 1–1½ CUPS (240–360 ML)

Ingredients

2 tbsp (5 g) horehound (*Marrubium vulgare*) leaf

1 tbsp (7 g) elecampane (*Inula helenium*) root

1 tbsp (2 g) plantain (*Plantago* spp.) leaf

1 cup (240 mL) water

½ cup (120 mL) raw honey

½ cup (120 mL) white pine (*Pinus strobus*) needle tincture (optional)

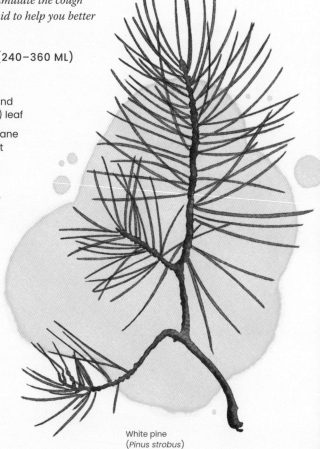

White pine
(*Pinus strobus*)

Directions

1 Measure herbs and combine them together in a small saucepan. Pour 1 cup (240 mL) of water over the plant material, stirring the mixture well to fully saturate the herbs with water, and place a lid on the saucepan. Allow this mixture to sit for 12–24 hours, giving the harder plant parts time to soften, if desired.

2 When you are ready to make the syrup, place the saucepan on the stove, remove the lid, and bring the mixture to a boil over medium-high heat. When the water comes to a boil, immediately reduce the heat to bring the mixture to a simmer and hold it there until the water level has reduced by half—to ½ cup (120 mL)—to create a decoction.

3 Once the water level has reduced to ½ cup (120 mL), carefully strain the decoction through a fine-mesh sieve (lined with a few layers of cheesecloth to remove any plant material, if you wish). Press the herbs with the back of a spoon (or gather the edges of the cheesecloth to create a bundle and squeeze) to extract as much liquid as possible. Reserve the decocted liquid in a clean glass measuring cup, adding more water, if needed, to bring the total volume of liquid up to ½ cup (120 mL), and compost the used plant material.

4 Allow the liquid to cool slightly before adding ½ cup (120 mL) of raw honey and ½ cup (120 mL) of tincture, if using. Stir well to combine and transfer to a labeled glass storage container. Cap and store for future use.

Usage

Take 1–2 tsp (5–10 mL) every 2–4 hours.

Storage & Shelf-life

Store in a cool, dark location. Use syrups made without a tincture within 3–4 weeks and use syrups made with a tincture within 12 months before making a fresh batch.

DIGEST–EASE PASTILLES

Support digestion after a heavy meal by eating one of these tasty lozenges. These powerhouse herbal pastilles are packed with botanicals to help support healthy digestion after a meal by easing cramps, gas, and bloating.

YIELD: VARIES

Ingredients

2 parts fennel (*Foeniculum vulgare*) seed powder

1 part ginger (*Zingiber officinale*) rhizome powder

½ part cinnamon (*Cinnamomum verum*) bark powder

½ part cardamom (*Elettaria cardamomum*) seed powder

Raw honey

Extra cinnamon (*Cinnamomum verum*) bark or fennel (*Foeniculum vulgare*) seed powder (for coating)

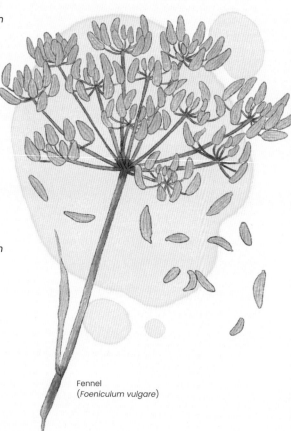

Fennel
(*Foeniculum vulgare*)

Directions

1 Begin by placing a small amount of each individual herb in a coffee grinder to grind into a powder. Sift the powder through a fine-mesh sieve, reserving the fine powder in a clean bowl (one bowl for each herbal powder) and composting the larger plant material that remains in the sieve.

2 When you are ready to make the pastilles, choose the measurement you'd like to use for your part and measure each herbal powder, combining them together in a large mixing bowl.

3 Add a small amount of honey to the powder and mix until a stiff dough forms. Adjust for consistency by adding more herbal powder to create a stiffer dough or more honey for a softer dough.

4 Once the dough is at the correct consistency to roll out little balls (pastilles), pinch off small pieces of dough and roll them into dime-sized balls. Transfer the dough balls into herbal powder to coat them. Cinnamon and fennel are tasty, but any flavorful herbal powder will work. Dust the dough balls in the coating powder and transfer them to a labeled glass storage container. Add some additional coating powder to the container to keep the pastilles from sticking to one another. Cap and store for future use.

Usage

Take 1 pastille after a heavy meal, letting it slowly dissolve in your mouth.

Storage & Shelf-life

Store in a cool, dark location. Use within 6 months before making a fresh batch.

Tip

• To make your own powders, place dried plant material, one herb at a time, in a coffee grinder. Set the grinder to a fine setting and grind for 30–60 seconds. Sift the ground plant material through a fine-mesh sieve, reserving the fine powder in a bowl and composting the coarse plant material that remains in the sieve.

Gut Restore Tea

Whether you've just recovered from a bought of diarrhea or you're concerned about the permeability of your intestinal lining (leaky gut, is that you?), you can show some love and care for your digestive tract by utilizing herbs that help tighten and tone tissues of the gut lining, stimulate tissue regeneration, soothe irritation, and ease inflammation.

YIELD: 1 CUP (240 ML)

Ingredients

1 cup (240 mL) water

1 tbsp (1–2 g) Gut Restore tea blend (below)

Raw honey, to taste (optional)

Gut Restore Tea Blend:

3 parts red raspberry (*Rubus* spp.) leaf

2 parts plantain (*Plantago* spp.) leaf

2 parts calendula (*Calendula officinalis*) flower

2 parts chamomile (*Matricaria chamomilla*) flower

1 part peppermint (*Mentha* x *piperita*) leaf

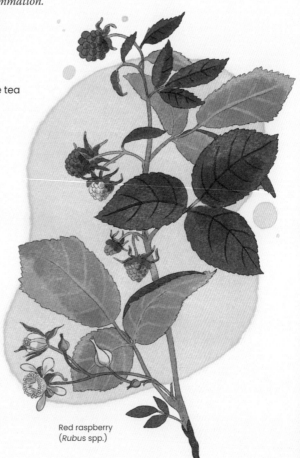

Red raspberry
(*Rubus* spp.)

Directions

1 Start by blending your Gut Restore tea blend together. Measure out each herb individually and combine them in a large mixing bowl, stirring the herbs well to fully blend them together. Transfer this tea blend to a labeled glass storage container. Cap and store for future use.

2 When you are ready to make your tea, bring 1 cup (240 mL) of water to a boil using a kettle or a small saucepan over medium-high heat. As soon as the water comes to a boil, remove it from the heat.

3 While the water is coming to a boil, place 1 tbsp of Gut Restore tea blend in a glass canning jar.

4 Pour 1 cup (240 mL) of boiled water over the plant material, cap, and set aside to infuse for 3–5 minutes.

5 When time is up, carefully strain the mixture through a fine-mesh sieve lined with an unbleached coffee filter to remove any fine particles. Press the herbs with the back of a spoon (or gather the edges of the coffee filter to create a bundle and gently squeeze) to extract as much liquid as possible. Reserve the liquid in a clean, heat-proof mug or glass canning jar and compost the used plant material. Sweeten with raw honey, if desired.

Usage

Drink up to 3 cups (720 mL) a day, hot or cold.

Storage & Shelf-life

Store tea blend in a cool, dark location. Use within 12 months before making a fresh batch.

Tip

• Make a whole day's worth of tea at once and store the extra tea in the refrigerator until you're ready to drink it. Use within 24 hours before making a fresh batch.

Raspberry leaf is a wonderful astringent herb that helps to tighten and strengthen tissues that have lost their tone. There are several species of raspberry that can be used interchangeably from red raspberry to black raspberry. So the next time you're out and about, keep an eye out for wild raspberries. The berries aren't the only useful part of the plant!

Move It Herb Bites

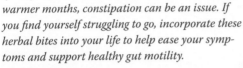

Not being able to go to the bathroom is no fun. Oftentimes in the cooler months of the year, when our diets become heavier and we move less than we do in warmer months, constipation can be an issue. If you find yourself struggling to go, incorporate these herbal bites into your life to help ease your symptoms and support healthy gut motility.

YIELD: 16 BITES

Ingredients

1 tbsp (12 g) flax seed, ground

1 tbsp (12 g) chia seed, ground

¼ cup (31 g) slippery elm (*Ulmus rubra*) powder**

¼ cup (60 mL) honey

2 tbsp (35 g) nut butter

2 tbsp (28 g) coconut oil

2 tbsp (16 g) triphala powder

Cinnamon (*Cinnamomum* spp.) powder (for coating)

** sustainably sourced only

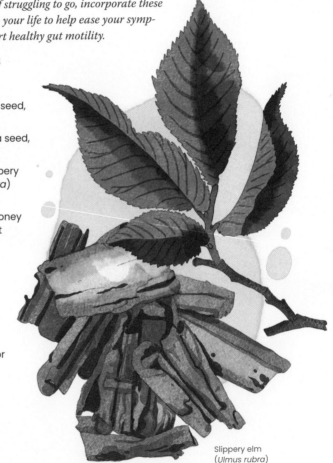

Slippery elm
(*Ulmus rubra*)

Directions

1 Measure flax and chia seeds and place them in a coffee grinder to grind into a powder. Transfer seed powders to a large bowl.

2 Measure all other ingredients and add to the bowl. Mix until a stiff dough forms. Adjust for consistency by adding more herbal powder to create a stiffer dough or more honey for a softer dough.

3 Once the dough is at the correct consistency to roll into balls, pinch off large pieces of dough and roll into tablespoon-sized balls. Transfer the dough balls into herbal powder to coat them. Dust the dough balls in the coating powder and transfer them to a labeled glass storage container. Add some additional coating powder to the container to keep the dough balls from sticking to one another. Cap and store for future use.

Usage

Eat 1–2 herb bites 3 times a day, along with other supportive lifestyle changes, until symptoms reside.

Storage & Shelf-life

Store in the refrigerator. Use within 2–3 weeks before making a fresh batch.

Tip

• Change up your herbal coating powder to vary the flavor of these herb bites. Choose from any flavorful herb, such as cinnamon, cardamom, fennel, licorice, peppermint, spearmint, etc.

Triphala means "three fruits," and it's the combination of equal parts amalaki (*Emblica officinalis*), bibitaki (*Terminalia bellerica*), and haritaki (*Terminalia chebula*) fruits (commonly know as amla, beleric myrobalan, and black myrobalan), which are dried, powdered, and blended together. This blend is a classic Ayurvedic approach to easing constipation with regular use.

WINTER

Winter, a season of stillness and rest for the plant world and for the herbalist, invites us to embrace the warmth of shared moments by the fire, cherish the company of loved ones, and find comfort in the simplicity of life's quiet joys. It is a season that teaches resilience, as life lies dormant beneath the surface, gathering strength for the inevitable rebirth that awaits in the coming spring.

While mostly a slow season where foraging is concerned, winter is a time when I like to sit back and take a moment to appreciate all the effort I have put into tending the earth and caring for my family during the previous seasons. At this point in the year's cycle, I find myself with an apothecary stocked full of botanicals from the year's harvest, waiting to be called upon as needed, and a natural medicine cabinet filled with preparations and formulations to see my family through the winter months. Nature's provision and my diligent preparation throughout the year allow me ample time to rest my mind and body, nourish myself, spend time with loved ones, and reflect on the blessings and lessons learned over the past year.

Depending on location and temperature, it is possible to find some herbs to forage in this season. While most plants lie dormant until spring when warmer temperatures return, there are some abundant botanicals available during winter. Conifer needles and resins can be gathered all season long from certain varieties of cedar (*Cedrus* spp.), fir (*Abies* spp.), hemlock (*Tsuga* spp.), juniper (*Juniperus* spp.), pine (*Pinus* spp.), and spruce (*Picea* spp.). Flavorful roots, such as sassafras (*Sassafras albidum*), should be harvested in winter when the sap is concentrated in the roots, giving them more flavor. Evergreen herbs, such as rosemary (*Salvia rosmarinus*), thyme (*Thymus vulgaris*), and wintergreen (*Gaultheria procumbens*) can also be harvested continually throughout the winter season.

Winter provides a time of stillness where we can rest, quiet the mind and body, and take time to relax and restore ourselves for the next cycle of increased energy. One way we can support the body during this time is to continue eating warm, nourishing foods, such as soups and stews, along-side roasted and braised vegetables, meats, beans, and grains. We can also add warm spices to meals and hot drinks, which aid digestion, and incorporate herbs high in minerals into our foods and drinks to support the kidneys and provide nourishment to the tissues.

In winter, our focus remains on our immune and endocrine systems, working to keep them strong and healthy. However, this season, spices and aromatics play a more prominent role in the apothecary, as well as herbs that help relax the mind and body and lift the spirits. Depending on location, winter can be a long season, so mood support and warming botanicals can help us meet many of our health and wellness needs.

Here, you will find several issues one might face during winter, along with supportive recipes and remedies to see you through this slow, dark season.

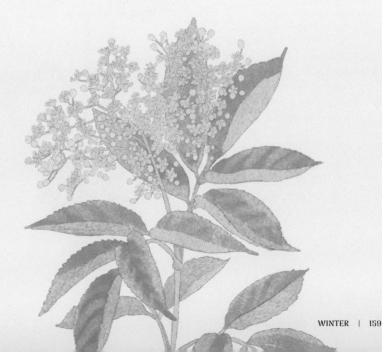

BRIGHTER DAYS AHEAD TINCTURE

The dark, cold days of winter can sometimes feel never-ending, especially after the holidays have passed and the festivities of the season are gone. Come the new year, it's easy to find oneself longing for the brighter, warmer days of spring, and it is here where our mood-supportive plant allies shine and offer a glimpse of brighter days ahead.

YIELD: VARIES

Ingredients

3 parts lemon balm (*Melissa officinalis*) aerial parts tincture or glycerite

2 parts tulsi (*Ocimum tenuiflorum*) aerial parts tincture or glycerite

1 part hawthorn (*Crataegus* spp.) berry tincture or glycerite

½ part rose (*Rosa* spp.) petal tincture or glycerite

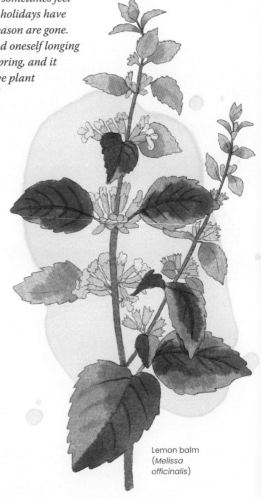

Lemon balm (*Melissa officinalis*)

Directions

1 Make individual tinctures or glycerites following directions on pages 35–39.

2 When you are ready to create the tincture or glycerite blend, begin by choosing the measurement you'd like to use for your part.

3 Measure out each tincture or glycerite individually before combining them in a clean, labeled glass storage container. Cap and store for future use.

Usage

Take ½–1 tsp (2.5–5 mL) 3 times a day until the spring equinox or the days begin to further brighten and warm up.

Storage & Shelf-life

Store in a cool, dark location. Use within 3–5 years before making a fresh batch.

Tip

- You can get a better extraction when tincturing herbs by blending the herbs and alcohol together in a high-speed blender for a couple of minutes before transferring the mixture to a glass canning jar. This increases the surface area of the herb and allows more of the solvent to come into contact with the plant material, thus increasing extraction.

Herbal Sunshine Tea

If the cold, dark days of winter have you moving slowly and feeling quite unmo-
tivated, why not try a warm cup of tea with a bit of a botanical pick-me-up?
This herbal blend is composed of botanicals that help improve mood and ease
feelings of anxiety or stress when used regularly. Say goodbye to the winter blues.
It's time to look to the sunny side of life! Note: This blend can be a tad on the bit-
ter side, so keep a close eye on your steep time. If you feel it's too bitter, you can
reduce the amount of hops (or leave them
out entirely) or bump the spearmint up
a touch.

YIELD: 1 CUP (240 ML)

Ingredients

1 cup (240 mL) water

1 tbsp (2 g) Herbal Sunshine
tea blend (below)

Raw honey, to taste
(optional)

Herbal Sunshine
Tea Blend:

3 parts hops
(*Humulus
lupulus*) strobile

2 parts lemon
balm (*Melissa
officinalis*) aerial
parts

1 part lemongrass
(*Cymbopogon
citratus*) leaf

1 part spearmint
(*Mentha spicata*) leaf

½ part ginger (*Zingiber officinale*) root

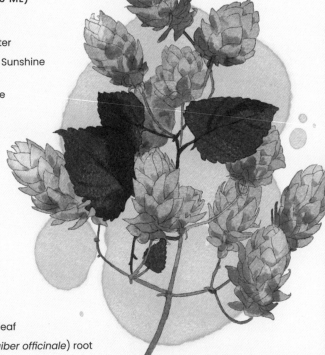

Hops
(*Humulus lupulus*)

Directions

1 Start by blending your Herbal Sunshine tea blend together. Measure out each herb individually and combine them in a large mixing bowl, stirring the herbs well to fully blend them together. Transfer this tea blend to a labeled glass storage container. Cap and store for future use.

2 When you are ready to make your tea, bring 1 cup of water to a boil using a kettle or a small saucepan over medium-high heat. As soon as the water comes to a boil, remove it from the heat.

3 While the water is coming to a boil, place 1 tbsp of Herbal Sunshine tea blend in a glass canning jar.

4 Pour 1 cup (240 mL) of boiled water over the plant material, cap, and set aside to infuse for 3–5 minutes.

5 When time is up, carefully strain the mixture through a fine-mesh sieve lined with an unbleached coffee filter to remove any fine particles. Press the herbs with the back of a spoon (or gather the edges of the coffee filter to create a bundle and gently squeeze) to extract as much liquid as possible. Reserve the liquid in a clean, heat-proof mug or glass canning jar and compost the used plant material. Sweeten with raw honey, if desired.

Usage

Drink up to 3 cups (720 mL) a day, hot or cold.

Storage & Shelf-life

Store tea blend in a cool, dark location. Use within 12 months before making a fresh batch.

The hops plant is a vigorous-growing vine that is easy to cultivate if you give it plenty of organic, nutrient-rich soil, a long growing season, and full sun. Because hops is a virulent vine and prefers to grow vertically, it needs to be planted somewhere where it has structure to support its weight, such as a trellis or fence. Be careful growing it near other plants, trees, or shrubs as it will use them for support and can strangle out tender plants.

Happy Heart Stress Glycerite

Winter can be a stress-filled season for many, whether due to the busyness of the holiday season, memories of a lost loved one, or the lack of warmth and light. While most of these stress triggers pass fairly quickly, for some, it can lead to ongoing feelings of anxiety and depression that negatively impact daily life. Thankfully, there are some herbs specific to strengthening the cardiovascular and nervous systems that can help lift the blues away, make the heart a bit happier, and ease feelings of stress as well. Plus, preparing them as a glycerite means they'll taste great, giving you a little treat to look forward to each day.

YIELD: 2 CUPS (480 ML)

Ingredients

¼ cup (35 g) hawthorn (*Crataegus* spp.) berry

¼ cup (4 g) rose (*Rosa* spp.) petal

2 tbsp (4 g) milky oat (*Avena sativa*) seed

2 tbsp (4 g) chamomile (*Matricaria chamomilla*) flower

1 tbsp (2 g) lemon balm (*Melissa officinalis*) aerial parts

¾ cup (180 mL) water

1¼ cups (300 mL) food-grade vegetable glycerin

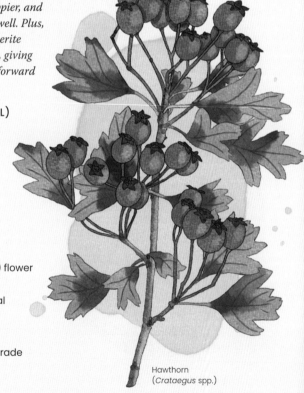

Hawthorn
(*Crataegus* spp.)

Directions

1 Measure ingredients and combine them together in a clean glass jar. All plant material should be covered with 2–3 inches (5–8 centimeters) of liquid as the plant material will expand after soaking up some of the liquid.

2 Place a piece of natural waxed paper between the jar and the lid to help prevent any chemical coating or corrosion on the lid from coming into contact with the contents inside the jar.

3 Label the jar and give it a shake to make sure the contents are mixed.

4 Place the jar on a seed-warming mat for two weeks. Be sure to gently shake the jar every day or two to keep the contents mixed up inside, as this will help give you a better extraction.

5 When your glycerite is finished, place a fine-mesh sieve (lined with a few layers of cheesecloth to remove plant material, if you wish) over a clean, dry glass container and carefully pour the mixture through it. Press the herbs with the back of a spoon (or gather the edges of the cheesecloth to create a bundle and gently squeeze) to extract as much liquid as possible. You can double strain the decanted liquid once more through a fine-mesh sieve lined with an unbleached coffee filter to further remove fine particles if you wish. Reserve the finished herb-infused oil in a clean, labeled glass storage container and compost the used plant material. Cap and store for future use.

Usage

Take 1–2 tsp (5–10 mL) 3 times a day.

Storage & Shelf-life

Store in a cool, dark location. Use within 2 years before making a fresh batch.

STRESS AWAY
AROMATHERAPY ROLLER

Sometimes, stress can feel overwhelming, and we need to hit the pause button and have a moment to ourselves. When this happens, don't forget to incorporate relaxing scents to help you destress even further. Scent is powerful and can help induce feelings of deep relaxation, not only for the mind but also for muscle tension in the body.

YIELD: 2 TSP (10 ML)

Ingredients

2 tsp (10 mL) olive oil

5 drops ylang ylang
(*Cananga odorata*)
essential oil

4 drops of lavender
(*Lavandula angustifolia*)
essential oil

3 drops of patchouli
(*Pogostemon cablin*)
essential oil

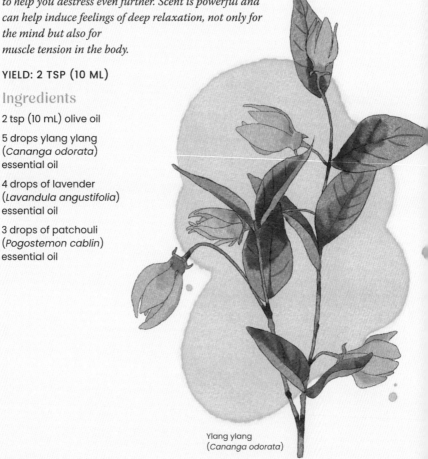

Ylang ylang
(*Cananga odorata*)

Directions

1 Using a small funnel, add the carrier oil and essential oils to a labeled glass roller bottle, creating a 6% dilution, which is the suggested dilution for aromatherapy blends used on small surface areas of the body during acute issues.

2 Insert the roller ball as instructed on the packaging. Cap and store for future use.

Usage

Apply a small amount of oil to the wrists, collarbone, neck, or behind the ears anytime you feel the need to ease feelings of stress.

Storage & Shelf-life

Store in a cool, dark location. Use within 1 year before making a fresh batch.

Tip

• Feel free to skip the carrier oil and place these essential oils in an aromatherapy inhaler instead.

Inhaling essential oils sends signals to the brain. These signals influence the nervous system and, therefore, have a physical and emotional impact on the body. In fact, when inhaled, odors follow a direct path to the brain's limbic system, which is made up of the amygdala and hippocampus, two tissues associated with emotion and memory. This is why scents have the power to evoke memories and elicit both positive and negative feelings, as well as why aromatherapy can be beneficial for easing stress and anxiety and promoting an overall sense of calm.

FEVER EASE TEA

Fevers, while a vital and necessary part of immune function, are no fun. Not only do they make one feel terrible, but sometimes they reach uncomfortably high temperatures and can cause a bit more concern. Thankfully, we have some herbal allies that can help support the body when infection is present and help to gently cool the body a touch at the same time.

YIELD: 1 CUP (240 ML)

Ingredients

1 cup (240 mL) water

1 tbsp (1–2 g) Fever Ease tea blend (below)

Raw honey, to taste (optional)

Fever Ease Tea Blend:

2 parts elder (*Sambucus nigra, S. canadensis*) flower

2 parts catnip (*Nepeta cataria*) aerial parts

1 part spearmint (*Mentha spicata*) leaf

1 part yarrow (*Achillea millefolium*) aerial parts

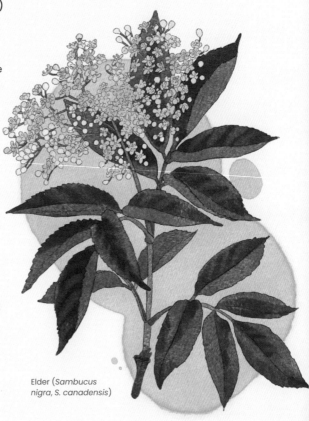

Elder (*Sambucus nigra, S. canadensis*)

Directions

1 Start by blending your Fever Ease tea blend together. Measure out each herb individually and combine them in a large mixing bowl, stirring the herbs well to fully blend them together. Transfer this tea blend to a labeled glass storage container. Cap and store for future use.

2 When you are ready to make your tea, bring 1 cup of water to a boil using a kettle or a small saucepan over medium-high heat. As soon as the water comes to a boil, remove it from the heat.

3 While the water is coming to a boil, place 1 tbsp of Fever Ease tea blend in a glass canning jar.

4 Pour 1 cup (240 mL) of boiled water over the plant material, cap, and set aside to infuse for 3–5 minutes.

5 When time is up, carefully strain the mixture through a fine-mesh sieve lined with an unbleached coffee filter to remove any fine particles. Press the herbs with the back of a spoon (or gather the edges of the coffee filter to create a bundle and gently squeeze) to extract as much liquid as possible. Reserve the liquid in a clean, heat-proof mug or glass canning jar and compost the used plant material. Sweeten with raw honey, if desired.

Usage

Drink ¼ cup (60 mL) of warmed tea every 30 minutes.

Storage & Shelf-life

Store tea blend in a cool, dark location. Use within 12 months before making a fresh batch.

Tip

• Be sure to drink this tea hot if you want to benefit from this blend's fever-easing properties. The diaphoretic action of herbs works best with hot liquid.

WARMING WINTERGREEN FOOT BATH

Whether you are chilled to the bone or supporting the body in reaching a higher temperature to ward off a cold or the flu, botanical foot baths can be an effective, and perhaps enjoyable, way to accomplish that goal. Not only will the heat of the water warm the feet and work its way up the body, but the circulatory enhancing action of the herbs will help to get blood moving, increasing warmth as well. Plus, it smells great and your tired, achy feet will thank you!

YIELD: 2 CUPS (480 ML)

Ingredients

2 cups (480 mL) water

1 cup (24 g) wintergreen (*Gaultheria procumbens*) leaf

½ cup (112 g) fresh ginger (*Zingiber officinale*) rhizome, grated

¼ cup (20 g) rosemary (*Salvia rosmarinus*) leaf

¼ cup (12 g) thyme (*Thymus vulgaris*) aerial parts

½ cup (NOTE g) Epsom salt

Directions

1 Bring water to a boil in a saucepan over medium-high heat.

2 While water is coming to a boil, measure out the herbs and combine them in a bowl. Set this aside until the water boils.

3 When the water boils, turn the heat off, add the herbs to the water in the saucepan, and stir them to combine with the water. Place a lid on the saucepan and allow this to steep for 30 minutes.

4 When time is up, strain the mixture through a fine-mesh sieve into a large pot or container—one that is big enough for both feet to fit into at the same time. Compost the herbs and mix Epsom salt into the water, stirring until fully dissolved.

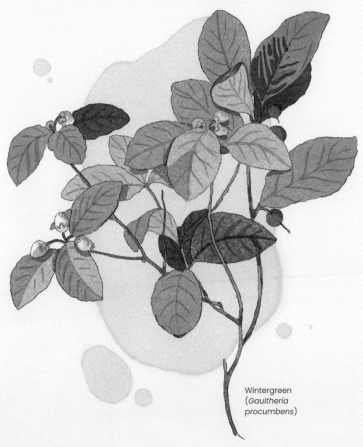

Wintergreen
(*Gaultheria procumbens*)

Usage

Soak the feet anytime you want to warm the body up a bit. Make sure the water is hot (but not so hot that it will burn the skin) before placing your feet in it. Soak your feet for 20–30 minutes.

Storage & Shelf-life

Store extras in the refrigerator for no more than 24 hours before making a fresh batch.

Spicy Salve

Sore muscles and stiff, achy joints can be common complaints during the colder months of the year, as well as cold hands and feet, so why not bring a little more warmth to these areas with a warming salve made from common kitchen spices? When gently massaged into the skin, this salve will help to bring added warmth to the tissues, increase circulation, and ease pain and stiffness.

YIELD: ½–1 CUP (120–240 ML)

Ingredients

1 tbsp (15 g) cayenne (*Capsicum annuum*) fruit

1 tbsp (6 g) ginger (*Zingiber officinale*) rhizome

1 tbsp (6 g) clove (*Syzygium aromaticum*) bud

1¼ tsp (3 g) black pepper (*Piper nigrum*) fruit

½–1 cup (120–240 ml) olive oil

¼–½ cup (28–56 g) beeswax, grated or pastille

12-24 drops of cinnamon (*Cinnamomum zeylanicum*) leaf essential oil (optional)

Cayenne
(*Capsicum annuum*)

Directions

1 Measure all ingredients and follow the steps for the quick or slow herb-infused oil method on pages 32–34.

2 When your oil is finished, place a fine-mesh sieve (lined with a few layers of cheesecloth to remove plant material, if you wish) over a clean, dry glass container and carefully pour the mixture through it. Press the herbs with the back of a spoon (or gather the edges of the cheesecloth to create a bundle and gently squeeze) to extract as much liquid as possible. You can double strain the decanted liquid once more through a fine-mesh sieve lined with an unbleached coffee filter to further remove fine particles if you wish and compost the used plant material.

3 When you are ready to make the salve, use a glass measuring cup or graduated cylinder to measure the amount of herb-infused oil you have. If needed, add more olive oil to bring the total volume of oil back up to the amount you started with: ½–1 cup (120–240 mL).

4 Measure out ¼ cup (28 g) of beeswax for every ½ cup (120 mL) of herb-infused oil you have. Place the beeswax into a clean saucepan, and heat it over medium-low heat until it has melted.

5 Turn the heat to low and pour the herb-infused oil into the saucepan alongside the melted beeswax. Carefully mix the two together until they're thoroughly combined.

6 Test the consistency of the salve by dipping a spoon in the mixture and letting it cool for a few minutes before touching it to get a feel for the final consistency. The goal is for the texture to be soft and easy to press. If the mixture is too hard, add a bit more oil. If the mixture is too soft, add another 1 tbsp (7 g) of beeswax. Be sure to go slow and make small adjustments, testing after each addition and repeating until you get the salve to the desired consistency.

7 Remove the saucepan from the heat and carefully transfer the mixture to a labeled tin or glass storage container.

8 If using, add 12 drops of cinnamon essential oil for every ½ cup (120 mL) of herb-infused oil to create a 0.5% dilution, which is the suggested dilution for strong essential oils used on small surface areas of the body. Stir the mixture with a toothpick and allow it to cool completely. Once cool, cap and store for future use.

Usage

Gently massage a small amount of salve into the skin as often as needed. For external use only!

Storage & Shelf-life

Store in a cool, dark location. Use within 12 months before making a fresh batch.

Tip

- To test the consistency of your salve before transferring it to a storage container, dip a spoon in the liquid mixture and place it in the refrigerator to cool quickly. If the salve is too soft, add a bit more wax to the saucepan. If the salve is too hard, add a bit more of the reserved herb-infused oil. Repeat the test until you get the consistency you desire, and then transfer to your storage container.

Spices are wonderful botanicals for easing pain and stiffness in the muscles and joints. They work by irritating the skin's surface, which dilates the blood vessels under the skin, allowing more blood flow to the region. Increased blood flow helps ease pain and inflammation and flush toxins and debris (like dead cells) from the area. Spices that are on the fresher side will work best as they will have retained more of their aromatic compounds. Keep your spices in well-sealed containers away from heat and light and only purchase what you can use within 6–12 months for maximum freshness and potency.

WINTER WOODLANDS SALVE

If winter has you down and out with a cold and suffering from sinus congestion, the invigorating scents of spruce and cedar needles can help not only support the immune system but also help you to feel as if you're breathing much easier. Paired with soothing calendula to calm and restore dry, irritated skin around the nose, this salve is a great way to experience the comforting embrace of the forest and breathe easier amid the winter chill. It also makes for a great way to reverse dry, chapped lips too!

YIELD: ½–1 CUP (120–240 ML)

Ingredients

½ cup (16 g) spruce (*Picea* spp.) needles

½ cup (7 g) calendula (*Calendula officinalis*) flower

1 tbsp (5 g) rosemary (*Salvia rosmarinus*) leaf

2 tbsp (4 g) peppermint (*Mentha* x *piperita*) leaf

½–1 cup (120–240 mL) olive oil

¼–½ cup (28–56 g) beeswax, grated or pastille

72–144 drops of pine (*Pinus* spp.) essential oil (optional)

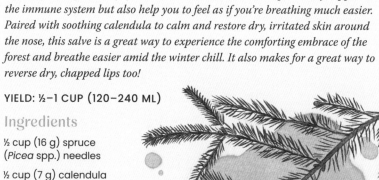

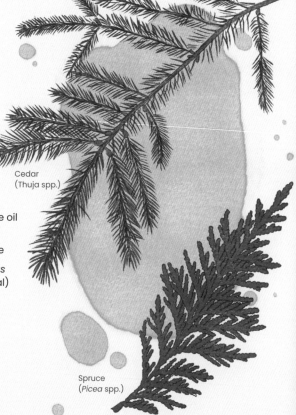

Cedar
(Thuja spp.)

Spruce
(*Picea* spp.)

Directions

1 Wearing protective gloves, gather enough fresh spruce needles by plucking the needles directly off the branches.

2 Measure all ingredients and follow the steps for the quick or slow herb-infused oil method on pages 32–34.

3 When your oil is finished, place a fine-mesh sieve (lined with a few layers of cheesecloth to remove plant material, if you wish) over a clean, dry glass container and carefully pour the mixture through it. Press the herbs with the back of a spoon (or gather the edges of the cheesecloth to create a bundle and gently squeeze) to extract as much liquid as possible. You can double strain the decanted liquid once more through a fine-mesh sieve lined with an unbleached coffee filter to further remove fine particles if you wish and compost the used plant material.

4 When you are ready to make the salve, use a glass measuring cup or graduated cylinder to measure the amount of herb-infused oil you have. If needed, add more olive oil to bring the total volume of oil back up to the amount you started with: ½–1 cup (120–240 mL).

5 Measure out ¼ cup (28 g) of beeswax for every ½ cup (120 mL) of herb-infused oil you have. Place the beeswax into a clean saucepan, and heat it over medium-low heat until it has melted.

6 Turn the heat to low and pour the herb-infused oil into the saucepan alongside the melted beeswax. Carefully mix the two together until they're thoroughly combined.

7 Test the consistency of the salve by dipping a spoon in the mixture and letting it cool for a few minutes before touching it to get a feel for the final consistency. The goal is for the texture to be firm. If the mixture is too hard, add a bit more oil. If the mixture is too soft, add another 1 tbsp (7 g) of beeswax. Be sure to go slow and make small adjustments, testing after each addition and repeating until you get the ointment to the desired consistency.

8 Remove the saucepan from the heat and carefully transfer the mixture to a labeled tin or glass storage container.

9 If using, add 72 drops of pine essential oil for every ½ cup (120 mL) of herb-infused oil to create a 3% dilution, which is the suggested dilution for products that cover a small surface area of the body. Stir the mixture with a toothpick. Once cool, cap and store for future use.

Usage

Apply a small amount of salve under the nose or to the chest and back (or other locations with dry, irritated skin), gently massaging into the skin, as often as needed.

Storage & Shelf-life

Store in a cool, dark location. Use within 12 months before making a fresh batch.

Conifer and mint plants contain a variety of volatile oil compounds. Certain compounds act on the nervous system to stimulate a cooling sensation that makes us feel as if there is more airflow moving through the nasal passages, therefore making us feel as if we can breathe better. Other volatile oil compounds are known to calm inflammation and swelling, thus helping ease sinus and nasal congestion.

BREATHE EASY SHOWER STEAMERS

When congestion is at its worst, the scent of cooling menthol and calming lavender can be just the thing you need for a bit of relief. Menthol helps you to feel like you can breathe better, and the scent of lavender relaxes the mind and body, the combination transforming your bathroom into an aromatherapeutic experience you will look forward to whether you're under the weather or simply want to relax.

YIELD: VARIES DEPENDING ON MOLD

Ingredients

2 cups (632 g) baking soda

1 cup (232 g) citric acid

½ cup (60 g) cornstarch

1 tbsp (12 g) menthol crystals

¼ cup (60 mL) grapeseed oil

22 drops of lavender (*Lavandula angustifolia*) essential oil

14 drops of eucalyptus (*Eucalyptus globulus*) essential oil

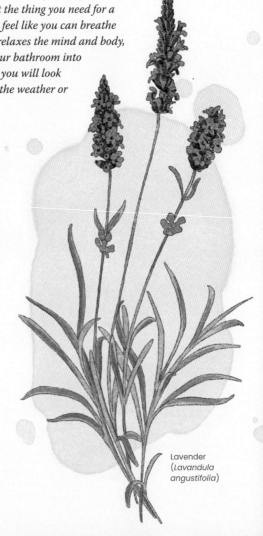

Lavender
(*Lavandula angustifolia*)

Directions

1 Begin by adding all powders to a glass bowl and carefully mixing to break up all clumps.

2 Place menthol crystals in a small saucepan and heat over medium-low heat to melt. Once melted, remove from heat and add grapeseed oil and essential oils, creating a 3% dilution, which is the suggested dilution for aromatic body care products that do not come into contact with the skin for prolonged periods of time. Stir well to combine.

3 Pour the oils into the powders and mix with a fork, being sure to break up any clumps that form.

4 While wearing gloves to protect your hands from the menthol and essential oils, you should be able to squeeze the mixture in your hand and have it hold together without crumbling. If it crumbles, put some witch hazel in a spray bottle and lightly spritz the powder while stirring until it will hold its shape when squeezed.

5 Press the powder into silicone molds, a small muffin tin, or free-form in your hand and set it aside to dry for 24 hours before transferring the shower steamers to a labeled glass storage container. Cap and store for future use.

Usage

Once your shower water is at your desired temperature, place the shower steamer on the shower floor just outside of the water stream. As it dissolves, it will release its aroma for you to inhale.

Storage & Shelf-life

Store in a dry, airtight location. Use within 2–3 months before making a fresh batch.

Tip

- Feel free to replace the oil in the recipe with 2 fl oz witch hazel, placing it in a spray bottle and gently spritzing the final powder mixture until it can hold its shape without crumbling when squeezed.

Get Well Honey

Garlic and ginger are two culinary herbs well-known for their immune-support-ive properties. These botanicals are commonly used fresh for bacterial and viral infections, particularly where respiratory infections are concerned. To make them more palatable and easy to use, mix them with a bit of raw honey to eat by the spoonful to ward off infections during the colder months of the year.

YIELD: ½–1 CUP (120–240 ML)

Ingredients

10–15 fresh garlic
(*Allium sativum*) cloves

2 tbsp (24 g) fresh ginger
(*Zingiber officinale*) rhizome

1 tbsp (8 g) Sweet Immunity Spice Blend (below)

½–1 cup (120–240 mL) raw honey

Sweet Immunity Spice Blend:

¼ cup (30 g) cinnamon
(*Cinnamomum verum*)
bark powder

1 tsp (2 g) ginger
(*Zingiber officinale*)
rhizome powder

½ tsp (1 g) nutmeg
(*Myristica fragrans*) seed
powder

½ tsp (1 g) cardamom
(*Elettaria cardamomum*)
seed powder

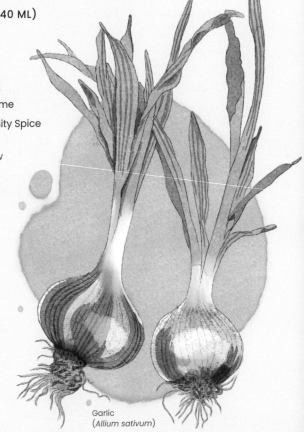

Garlic
(*Allium sativum*)

Directions

1 Remove the skin from 10–15 garlic cloves (approximately 1 bulb of garlic) and finely mince. Set this aside in a labeled glass storage container.

2 Grate or mince the ginger, adding it to the garlic in the glass storage container along with a tablespoon of the Sweet Immunity spice blend.

3 Add enough raw honey to cover the herbs in the container, stirring well to combine. Let this sit for 10 minutes to give the properties in the garlic time to activate.

4 Taste the mixture to see if you want to adjust the flavors. Add more fresh ginger if you'd like a bit more spice. Add more spice blend or honey to sweeten it up a bit. Add more garlic if you want to pack a stronger microbial punch. This is your opportunity to make it your own.

5 Cap and store for future use.

Usage

Take a spoonful of honey every 2–3 hours during acute bacterial or viral infections, doing your best to eat all of the herbs each day for best results.

Storage & Shelf-life

Store in the refrigerator and make a fresh batch every 1–2 days.

Tips

• Avoid using raw honey for children under 12 months of age. Instead, use maple syrup or food-grade vegetable glycerin.

• If you don't enjoy chewing the bits of garlic and ginger or swallowing them whole, you can blend the herbs and honey together in a personal blender to liquify the plant material and make it easier to take.

Allicin, the compound responsible for the characteristic odor and many of the health benefits associated with garlic, is activated when garlic cloves are chopped, crushed, or otherwise damaged, which triggers an enzymatic reaction that converts the precursor compound alliin into allicin. The process of allicin formation begins immediately upon crushing or chopping garlic, and it peaks within a few minutes. In addition to allicin, the health benefits of garlic are also attributed to other sulfur-containing compounds formed during the breakdown of allicin. These compounds may continue to develop and change over time, so it's a good idea to let garlic preparations sit for 10–20 minutes before using them. With that in mind, also know that allicin is unstable and can degrade over time, so consuming freshly chopped or crushed garlic may provide the most potent source of allicin and its related compounds.

RESPIRATORY RESCUE TINCTURE

When deep respiratory congestion or infection is present, this tincture recipe will truly feel like it is coming to the rescue. Filled with botanicals to thin mucous so it can be coughed up more easily while relaxing the smooth muscles of the bronchioles and working to deter microbes at the same time, this formula is a winter must-have.

YIELD: VARIES

Ingredients

4 parts usnea (*Usnea* spp.) lichen tincture or glycerite*

2 parts osha (*Ligusticum porteri*) root tincture or glycerite*

1 part echinacea (*Echinacea angustifolia, E. purpurea*) root tincture or glycerite**

1 part goldenseal (*Hydrastis canadensis*) root tincture or glycerite**

1 part licorice (*Glycyrrhiza glabra*) root tincture or glycerite

½ part wild cherry (*Prunus serotina*) bark tincture or glycerite

½ part skullcap (*Scutellaria lateriflora*) aerial parts tincture or glycerite

* sustainably sourced

** cultivated source

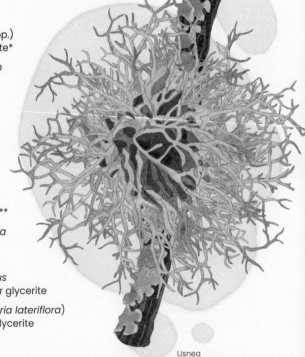

Usnea
(*Usnea* spp.)

Directions

1 Make individual tinctures and glycerites following directions on pages 35–39.

2 When you are ready to create the tincture or glycerite blend, begin by choosing the measurement you'd like to use for your part.

3 Measure out each tincture or glycerite individually before combining them in a clean, labeled glass storage container. Cap and store for future use.

Usage

Take 20–60 drops (1–3 mL) up to 6 times a day until symptoms reside.

Storage & Shelf-life

Store in a cool, dark location. Use within 3–5 years before making a fresh batch.

Usnea, also known as old man's beard, is a lichen—a combination of algae and fungi living synergistically together—that grows slowly on the branches of trees. It is highly prized for its ability to stimulate the immune system and keep microbes in balance. Usnea is difficult to cultivate and must therefore be sustainably sourced by gathering fallen pieces off the forest floor or broken branches after a storm.

WARMING WINTER OIL

Winter is tough on the skin, often leaving it dry and itchy. Massaging the skin daily with nourishing oils infused with warming botanicals can do wonders, not only for easing winter skin woes but for warming peripheral circulation as well. This herb-infused oil can be used as a daily protectant for the skin or as a deep massage oil for sore muscles.

YIELD: ½–1 CUP (120–240 ML)

Ingredients

3 tbsp (15 g) rosemary (*Salvia rosmarinus*) leaf

1 tbsp (8 g) juniper (*Juniperus* spp.) berry

1 tbsp (6 g) orange (*Citrus* spp.) peel

½–1 cup (120–240 mL) mustard oil

48–96 drops of sweet orange (*Citrus sinensis*) essential oil (optional)

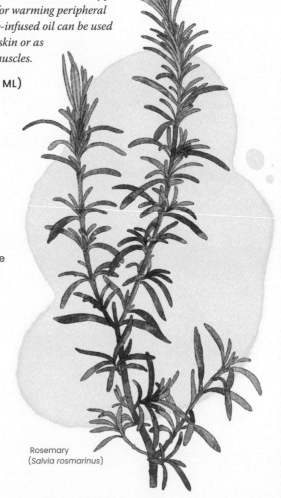

Rosemary
(*Salvia rosmarinus*)

Directions

1 Measure all ingredients and follow the steps for the quick or slow herb-infused oil method on pages 32–34.

2 When your oil is finished, place a fine-mesh sieve (lined with a few layers of cheesecloth to remove plant material, if you wish) over a clean, dry glass container and carefully pour the mixture through it. Press the herbs with the back of a spoon (or gather the edges of the cheesecloth to create a bundle and gently squeeze) to extract as much liquid as possible. You can double strain the decanted liquid once more through a fine-mesh sieve lined with an unbleached coffee filter to further remove fine particles if you wish and compost the used plant material.

3 Use a glass measuring cup or graduated cylinder to measure the amount of herb-infused oil you have. If needed, add more mustard oil to bring the total volume of oil back up to the amount you started with: ½–1 cup (120–240 mL).

4 If using, add 48 drops of sweet orange essential oil for every ½ cup (120 mL) of herb-infused oil to create a 2% dilution, which is the suggested dilution for body care products that cover a larger surface area of the body.

5 Mix well with a spoon. Transfer the finished oil to a labeled glass storage container and allow it to cool completely. Once cool, cap and store for future use.

Usage

Massage oil into dry skin as often as needed.

Storage & Shelf-life

Store in a cool, dark location. Use within 12 months before making a fresh batch.

Tip

• Don't have mustard oil on hand? You can make a DIY version by blending ½ cup (95 g) yellow and ½ cup (95 g) brown mustard seeds with 1 cup (240 mL) of olive oil in a high-speed blender for 2–3 minutes before filtering the mixture through a fine-mesh sieve (lined with a few layers of cheesecloth to remove plant material). Press the herbs with the back of a spoon (or gather the edges of the cheesecloth to create a bundle and gently squeeze) to extract as much liquid as possible. Double strain the decanted liquid once more through a fine-mesh sieve lined with an unbleached coffee filter to further remove fine particles and compost the used plant material.

Winter Wonderland Body Butter

Everyone needs a little self-care every now and then, especially during the winter months, and this decadent body butter is just the thing to provide a little extra luxury to your routine. Slather it on after a shower or long bath, or massage it into your skin at the end of a long day.

YIELD: 1 CUP (240 ML)

Ingredients

¼ cup (60 mL) coconut oil

¼ cup (60 mL) shea butter

¼ cup (60 mL) cocoa butter

¼ cup (60 mL) sweet almond oil

1 vanilla bean pod

48 drops of a conifer essential oil of your choice (optional)

1 tbsp (8 g) arrowroot powder

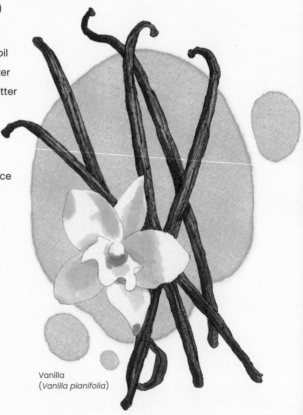

Vanilla
(*Vanilla planifolia*)

Directions

1 Gently heat coconut oil in a small saucepan until melted. Carefully measure out ¼ cup (60 mL) of oil and transfer it to a clean glass bowl. (Feel free to transfer the remaining melted coconut oil to another bowl to cool and harden before transferring it back to its storage container.) Repeat this process for the shea and cocoa butters, transferring ¼ cup (60 mL) of each melted butter into the bowl. Finally, add ¼ cup (60 mL) of sweet almond oil.

2 Transfer the bowl of melted liquid to the refrigerator to cool for 30–60 minutes until there is no longer a semi-liquid center.

3 While the liquid oils are cooling, slice 1 vanilla bean pod in half lengthwise and scrape the seeds out with a spoon. Set this aside in a small bowl.

4 Once the oil has cooled, remove the bowl from the refrigerator and use an immersion blender or electric mixer to whip the mixture on high for 5 minutes, periodically stopping to scrape the sides of the bowl. As you blend, the mixture will change color and begin to look light and fluffy.

5 Add vanilla bean seeds to the mixture and, if using, add 48 drops of a conifer essential oil to create a 1% dilution, which is the suggested dilution for body care products used on a large surface area of the body, along with arrowroot powder to help the body butter feel less greasy on your skin. Blend once more to thoroughly incorporate all ingredients.

6 Transfer the body butter to a labeled glass storage container. Cap and store for future use.

Usage

Apply a small amount to the skin, massaging it into the skin using small circular motions as often as you desire.

Storage & Shelf-life

Store in a cool, dark location. Use within 12 months before making a fresh batch.

Tip

• Don't throw the scraped vanilla pod away! Use it to make a vanilla-infused oil, vanilla paste, or vanilla extract.

ꟿIDWINTER APÉRITIF CORDIAL

In winter, we often find ourselves eating heavier, richer foods, so supporting digestion before a meal is beneficial in helping our digestive system properly digest the foods we eat. Bitter and carminative herbs can come to our aid in a supportive and delicious way when we incorporate them into cordials and enjoy a small amount before a heavy meal. Both bitter and carminative herbs are often high in volatile oils, which help relax our minds and the smooth muscle of the digestive tract, ease gas and bloating, and minimize cramping that is some-times associated with heavier meals of the winter season. It's a great idea to start this cordial after Thanksgiving so it's ready by the Winter Solstice.

YIELD: 3 CUPS (720 ML)

Ingredients

3 tbsp (24 g) gentian
(*Gentiana lutea*) root**

3 tbsp (20 g) orange
(*Citrus spp.*) peel

3 tbsp (18 g) fennel
(*Foeniculum vulgare*) seed

3 tbsp (15 g) rosemary
(*Salvia rosmarinus*) leaf

2 tbsp (12 g) ginger
(*Zingiber officinale*) rhizome

1 tbsp (8 g) dandelion
(*Taraxacum officinale*) root

2 cups (480 mL) brandy

½ cup (120 mL) raw honey

½ cup (120 mL) water

** cultivated source

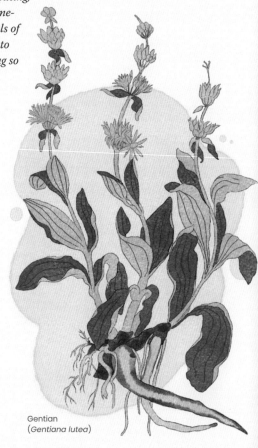

Gentian
(*Gentiana lutea*)

Directions

1 Measure each herb and combine them together in a quart-sized glass canning jar.

2 Pour 2 cups (480 mL) brandy over the plant material, and place a piece of natural waxed paper between the jar and the lid to protect the contents from any chemicals that are on the lid.

3 Label the jar and place it in a dark location for 4–6 weeks. Shake the jar every couple of days to keep the herbs and alcohol well-dispersed.

4 When time is up, carefully pour the mixture through a fine-mesh sieve (lined with a few layers of cheesecloth to remove any plant material, if you wish). Press the herbs with the back of a spoon (or gather the edges of the cheesecloth to create a bundle and squeeze) to extract as much liquid as possible and transfer the liquid to a bowl.

5 Measure out ½ cup (120 mL) of raw honey and ½ cup (120 mL) of water. Add these to the bowl with the herbal tincture and stir well to combine. Taste and add more honey if additional sweetness is desired.

6 Transfer the finished cordial to a clean, labeled glass storage container. Cap and store for future use.

Usage

Pour 2–4 tbsp (30–60 mL) into a glass. Sip 15–20 minutes before a heavy meal to support digestion and minimize the chance of gas, bloating, or cramping afterward.

Storage & Shelf-life

Store in a cool, dark location. Use within 12 months before making a fresh batch.

Harvest your own bitter orange peel by using a paring knife and cutting strips of the skin away from organic oranges before eating the juicy inner fruit. The white pith is quite nutritious and where the majority of the bitter properties lie, so be sure to leave some of the pith on the skin as you peel it. Transfer the peels to a dehydrator and dry on low heat until the peels dry up. You'll know they're completely dry when they bend and break easily.

Sweet Sleep Elixir

Getting a good night's sleep is vital to overall health. On nights when sleep doesn't come as easily as it does other nights, let the sleep-supportive properties of relaxing nervine and sedative herbs alongside raw honey help you drift off (or get back to) sleep. These ingredients help to ease the mind and body so it can fall asleep more easily, stay asleep longer, or fall back asleep after waking much faster.

YIELD: VARIES

Ingredients

4 parts passionflower (*Passiflora incarnata*) aerial parts tincture or glycerite

2 parts skullcap (*Scutellaria lateriflora*) aerial parts tincture or glycerite

2 parts valerian (*Valeriana officinalis*) root tincture or glycerite

1 part chamomile (*Matricaria chamomilla*) flower tincture or glycerite

9 parts raw honey

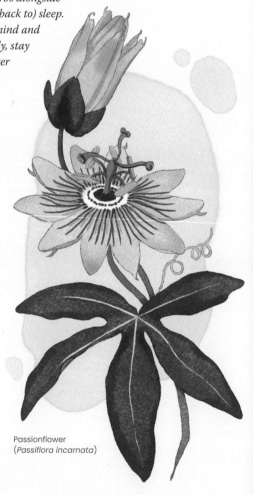

Passionflower
(*Passiflora incarnata*)

Directions

1 Make individual tinctures or glycerites following directions on pages 35–39.

2 When you are ready to create the tincture or glycerite blend, begin by choosing the measurement you'd like to use for your part.

3 Measure out each tincture or glycerite individually before combining them in a clean glass measuring cup or graduated cylinder.

4 Take note of the total volume of combined tinctures and add an equal amount of raw honey to sweeten the liquid and further support sleep. Stir well to combine. (If you are using glycerites, there is no need to add honey to this recipe.)

5 Transfer the elixir to a labeled glass storage container. Cap and store for future use.

Usage

Take anywhere from 1–3 tsp (5–15 mL) 30 minutes before bed or upon waking in the middle of the night.

Storage & Shelf-life

Store in a cool, dark location. Use within 1–3 years before making a fresh batch.

Honey contains tryptophan, which is an essential amino acid that is converted into melatonin—a hormone that helps relax and send sleep signals to the body. Because tryptophan is an essential amino acid and cannot be produced naturally in the body, supplementing with honey before bed is a great way to increase this essential nutrient in your diet.

INDEX

Q

Quease-Ease Syrup, 92–93
quick-heat herb-infused oil,
33–34

R

red raspberry leaf
    Gut Restore Tea,
        154–155
reishi mushroom
    Immune Tonic Broth
        Blend, 120–121
Respiratory Rescue
    Tincture, 186–187
rose hip
    High C Infusion,
        134–135
rose petal
    Brighter Days Ahead
        Tincture, 160–161
    Happy Heart Stress
        Glycerite, 164–165
    Sinus Soother Rinse,
        52–53
    tincture of, 40
rosemary
    Midwinter Apéritif
        Cordial, 192–193
    Scarborough Cider,
        122–124
    Warming Winter Oil,
        188–189
    Warming Wintergreen
        Foot Bath, 170–171
    Winter Woodlands
        Salve, 176–178

S

safety, 25–30
sage
    Oh! My Aching Head
        Tincture, 138–139

Scarborough Cider,
    122–124
    Sore Throat Pastilles,
        140–141
    Sore Throat Spray,
        74–75
    tincture of, 39, 40
    Up and Out Cough
        Syrup, 148–149
Scarborough Cider,
    122–124
sensitivities, herbal, 25–26
shea butter
    Winter Wonderland
        Body Butter, 190–191
Sinus Soother Rinse, 52–53
skullcap
    Respiratory Rescue
        Tincture, 186–187
    Splitting Headache
        Tincture, 108
    Sweet Sleep Elixir,
        194–195
    tincture of, 40
slippery elm
    Move It Herb Bites,
        156–157
Slow Down Styptic Powder,
    94
slow-heat herb-infused
    oil, 32
Sore Throat Pastilles,
    140–141
Sore Throat Spray, 74–75
spearmint
    Fever Ease Tea,
        168–169
    Herbal Sunshine Tea,
        162–163
Spicy Salve, 172–174
Splitting Headache
    Tincture, 108
Sprain Away Salve,
    114–116
Spring Allergy-Ease
    Infusion, 48–50

Spring Digestive Bitters,
    76–77
Spring Reset Chai Tea,
    46–47
spruce
    Winter Woodlands
        Salve, 176–178
St. John's wort
    Wound-a-Way Herbal
        Oil, 98–99
Stress Away Aromatherapy
    Roller, 166–167
substitutions, 22–23
Sunburn Spritzer, 84–85
supplies, sourcing, 16–18
sweet almond oil
    Winter Wonderland
        Body Butter, 190–191
sweet orange essential oil
    Warming Winter Oil,
        188–189
Sweet Sleep Elixir, 194–195

T

tea tree essential oil
    All-Purpose Herbal
        Ointment, 64–66
    Aromatic Earache
        Oil, 70
    Black Drawing Salve,
        72–73
    GOOT Ointment,
        142–144
    Wound-a-Way Herbal
        Oil, 98–99
thyme
    Immune Tonic Broth
        Blend, 120–121
    Scarborough Cider,
        122–124
    Warming Wintergreen
        Foot Bath, 170–171
tinctures, 34–38, 39–40
tissue affinities, 23

ACKNOWLEDGMENTS

To Susan Kopaka, thank you for gifting me my first herb book that night in the emergency room and for encouraging me to blend these two worlds together. To John Gallager, thank you for bringing so much herbal knowledge together in the Learning Herbs membership at such an affordable rate. To all the herbalists who said "yes" to sharing their wisdom through online courses, some of whom were Rosemary Gladstar, 7Song, Rosalee de la Forêt, jim mcdonald, Larken Bunce, all the instructors at Herbal Academy, and Sajah Popham—thank you from this small-town girl who didn't have access to local herbal teachers or schools. To Shoshanna Pearl and James Easling, thank you for investing in me by paying my way through my first formal herbal program with Herbal Academy and for giving me my first job as an herbalist. And to my Herbal Academy coworkers, thank you for all your support, encouragement, and guidance over the years. You all are the best team ever, and I wouldn't be the herbalist I am without you!

To my husband and boys, thank you for your never-ending support and encouragement on this journey; for always being up for a foraging trip, helping me make preparations in the kitchen, or listening to a new herbal tidbit or fact I want to share; for keeping all the plates spinning when I am busy working on a project or deadline; and for being so willing to follow my suggestions, even when you don't feel like it. You are the reason I do what I do.

Most importantly, to the one who created it all, thank you for being a lamp unto my feet and a light unto my path. To you, I give all the glory, honor, and praise.

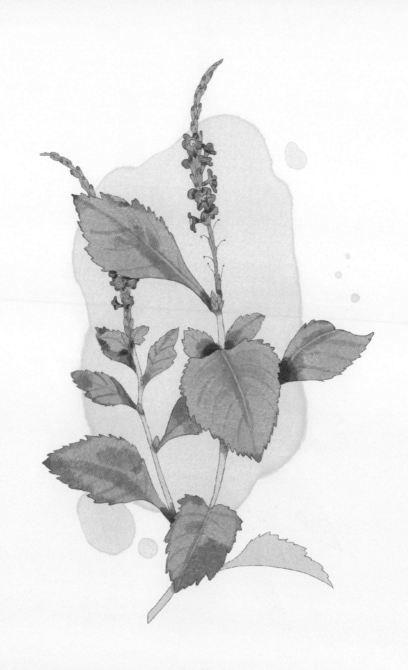

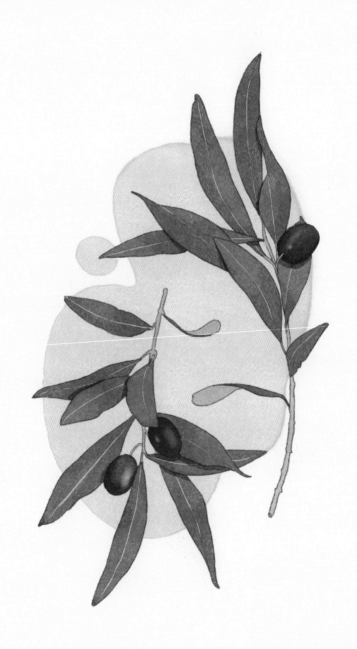

Author Bio

Meagan Visser is a registered nurse turned herbalist who lives with her husband and four sons in the beautiful southern Appalachian mountains. As a Staff Herbalist and Lead Herbalist Educator at Herbal Academy, Meagan brings a wealth of knowledge to her contributions, blending her medical background with timeless herbal wisdom. She is also the founder of Growing Up Herbal, a platform dedicated to natural living for families. When she's not teaching or crafting herbal preparations, Meagan enjoys homeschooling her children, gathering with friends and family, and spending time in her gardens, where she finds inspiration in the beauty of nature.

About Cider Mill Press Book Publishers

Good ideas ripen with time. From seed to harvest, Cider Mill Press brings fine reading, information, and entertainment together between the covers of its creatively crafted books. Our Cider Mill bears fruit twice a year, publishing a new crop of titles each spring and fall.

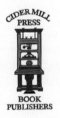

"Where Good Books Are Ready for Press"

501 Nelson Place
Nashville, Tennessee 37214

cidermillpress.com